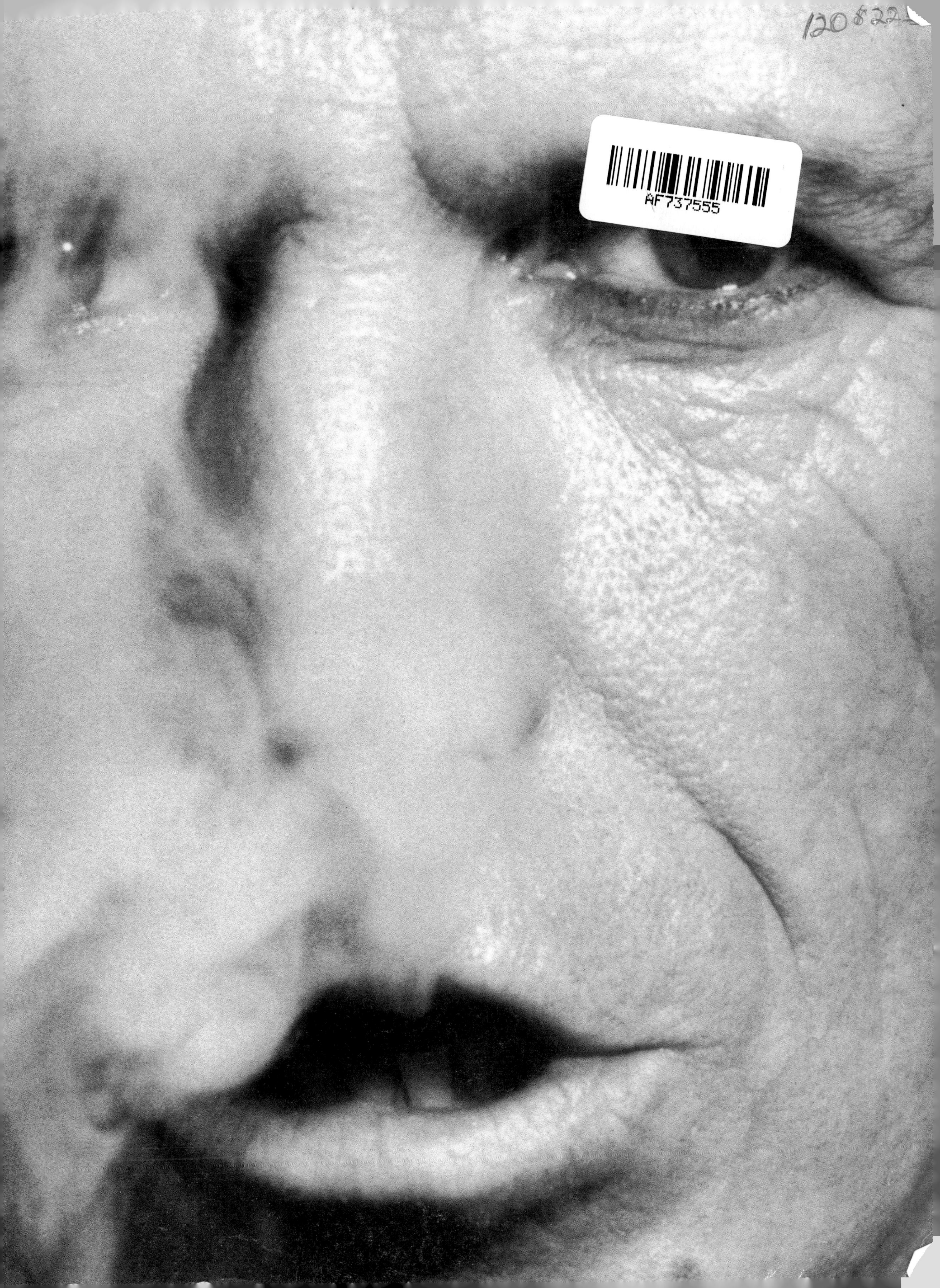

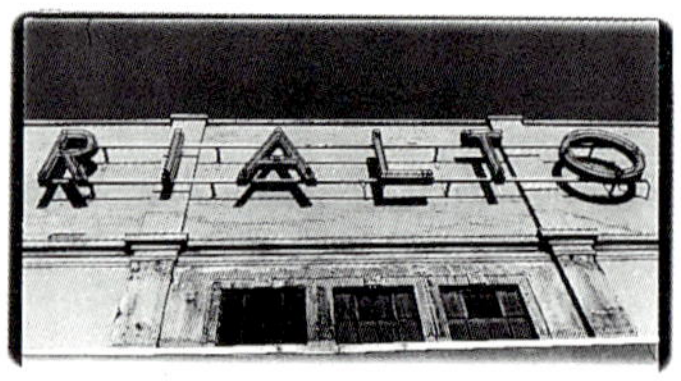

Raynes Park, '75

ACKNOWLEDGMENTS

For Their Invaluable Support And Assistance In Helping To Make This Book A Reality I Would Like To Thank:

Wilf Wright, Richard Bishop, Henry Rollins, Scarlet Page and Kazuyo Horie.

Black & White Printing:
Isgo & Baret Lepejian in Los Angeles
& Hugo Platt in London

Hand Tinting:
Phil Lemon

Halfin Photo:
Scarlet Page

Book Design:
Kathe Schreyer

And Thanks To
Pete Makowski, Mick Wall, and Chris Haskett
For Their Contributions To This Book.

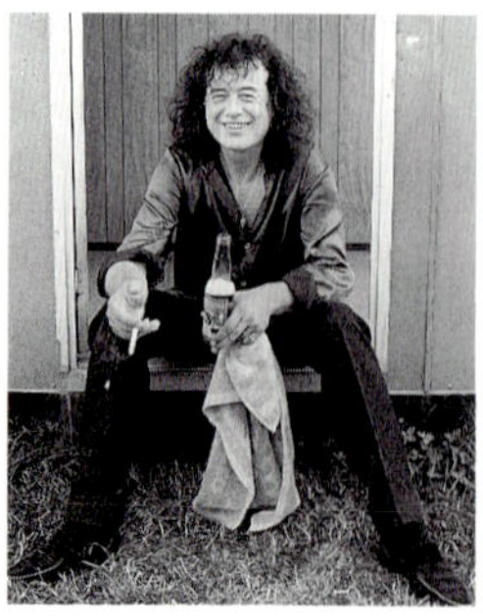

Jimmy Page
Glastonbury, June 25, 1995

120 #22

INTRODUCTION

"Working with Ross Halfin is as fun as shaving your head with a cheese grater while chewing on a cactus. He's not only the *biggest* pain in the ass on this planet, he's their leader. (He has assistants.) On tour, whenever his name is mentioned along with the fact that he's gracing us with his presence, our eyes light up (with hatred or fear of boredom) and we can't wait to wake up early for another brilliant adventurous photo session (standing in front of another white wall). But the most annoying thing of all is that we must put up with all this shit because he produces some of the most amazing shots ever!!

Luv,

James Hetfield
Metallica

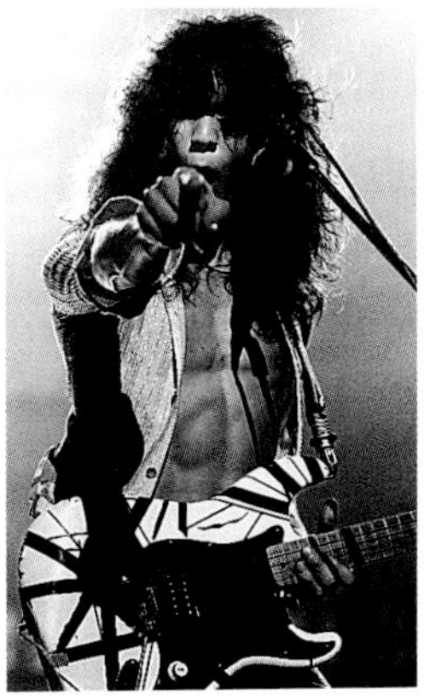

Eddie Van Halen
Rainbow Theater

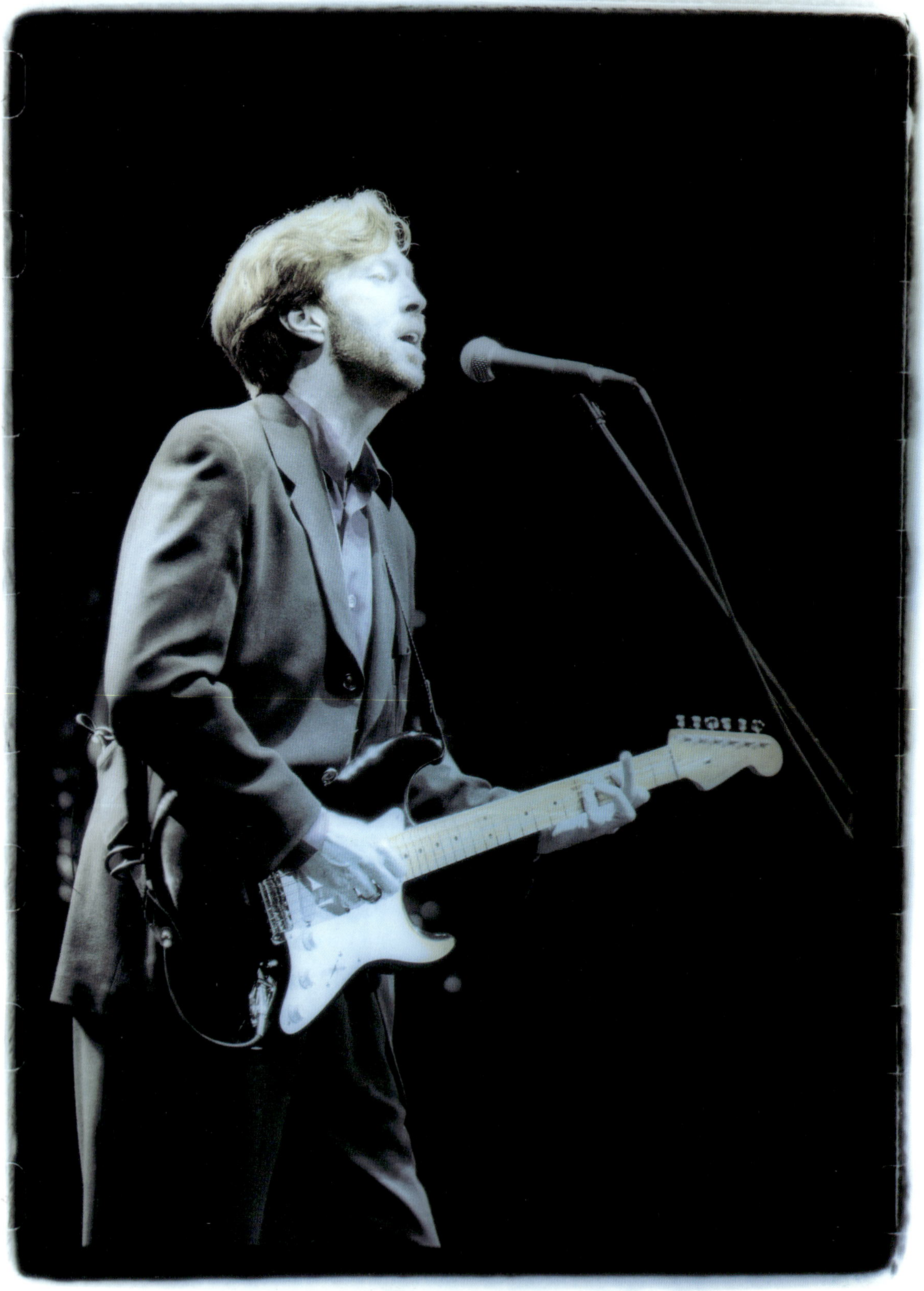

Eric Clapton
Albert Hall, London

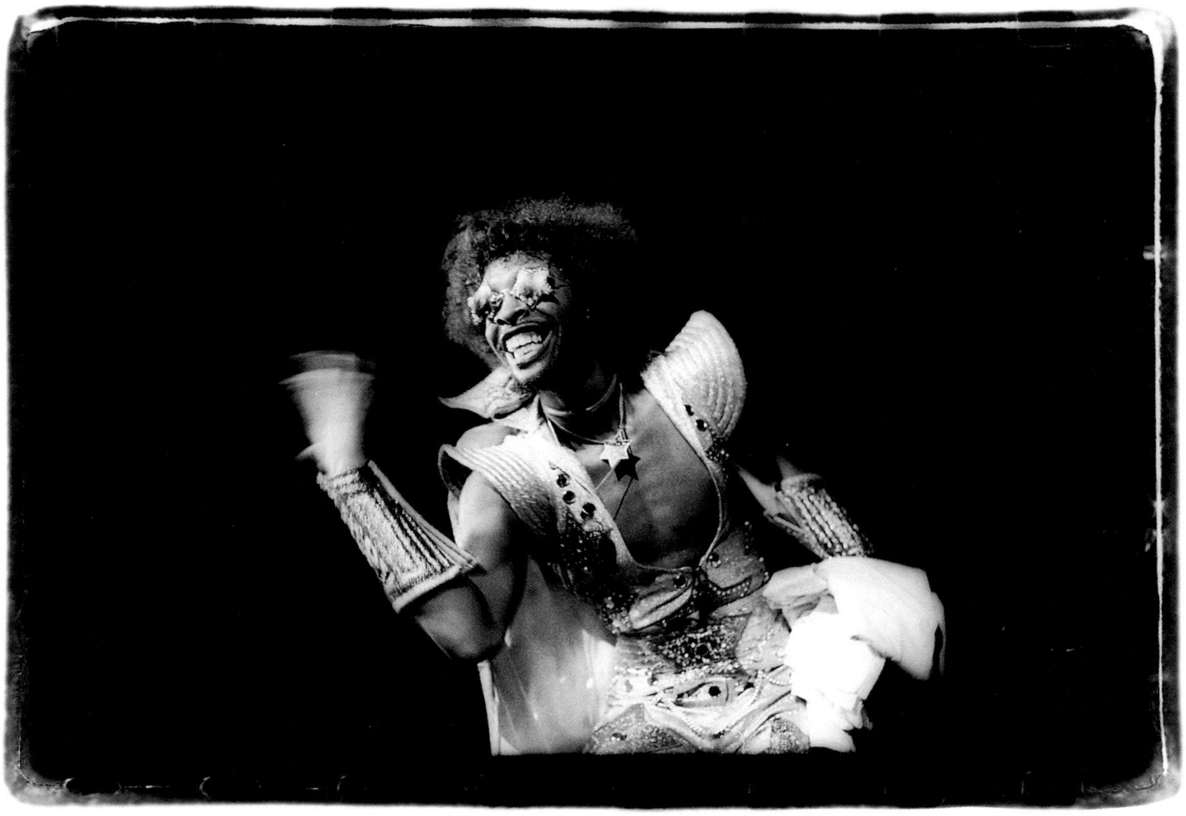

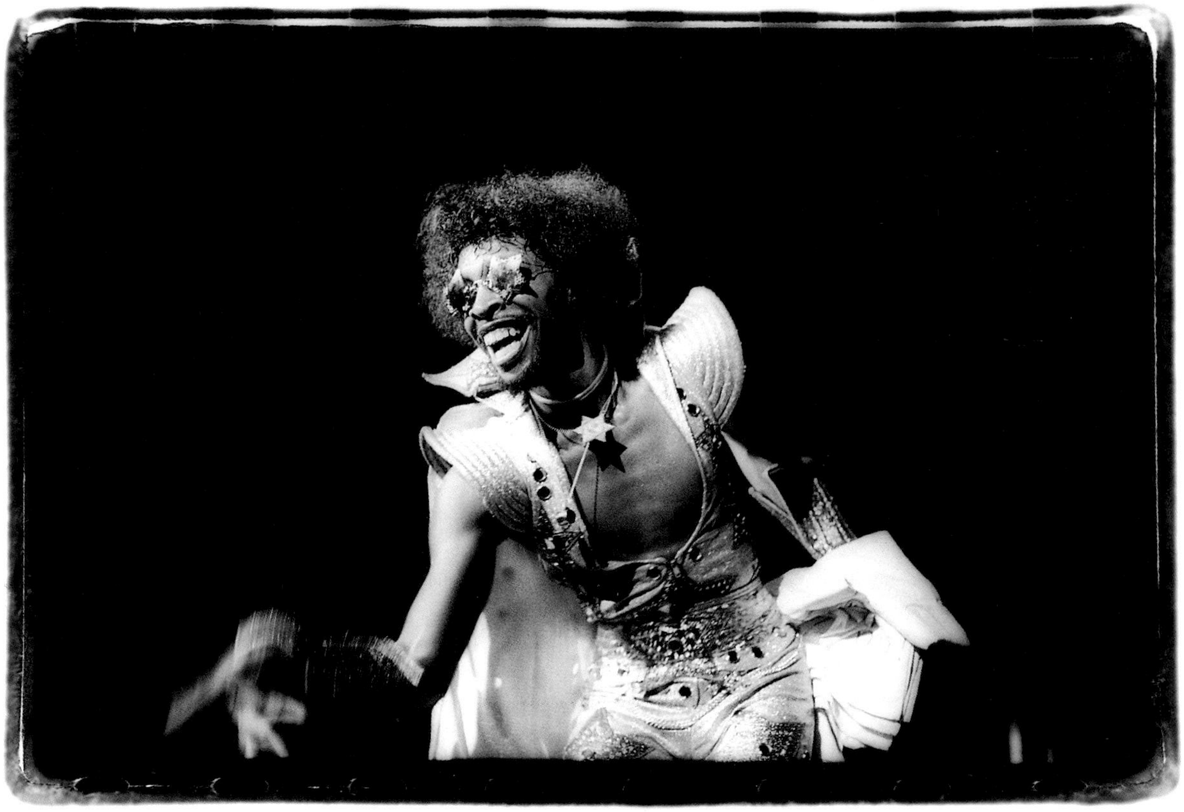

Bootsy
Hammersmith Odeon, London

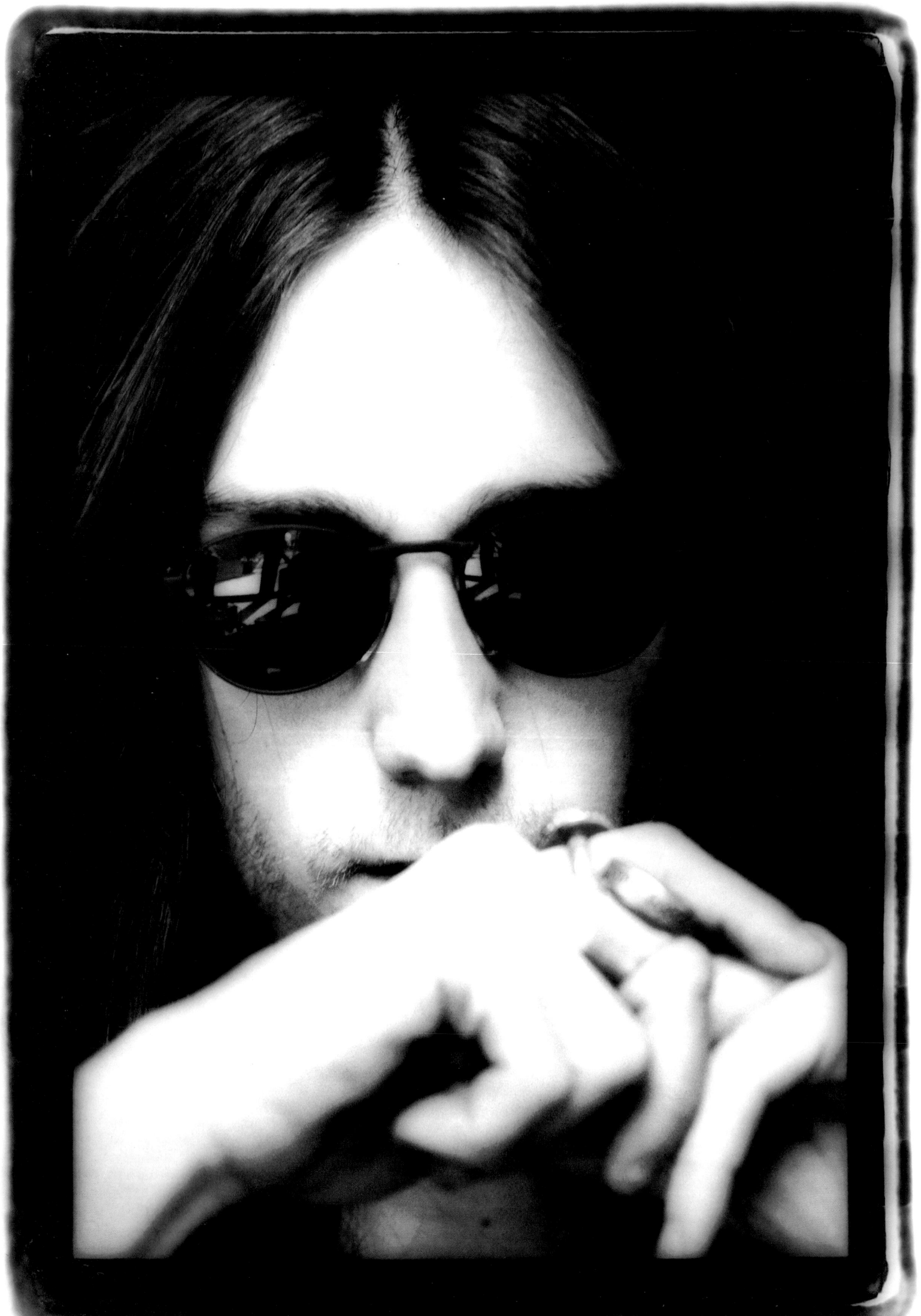

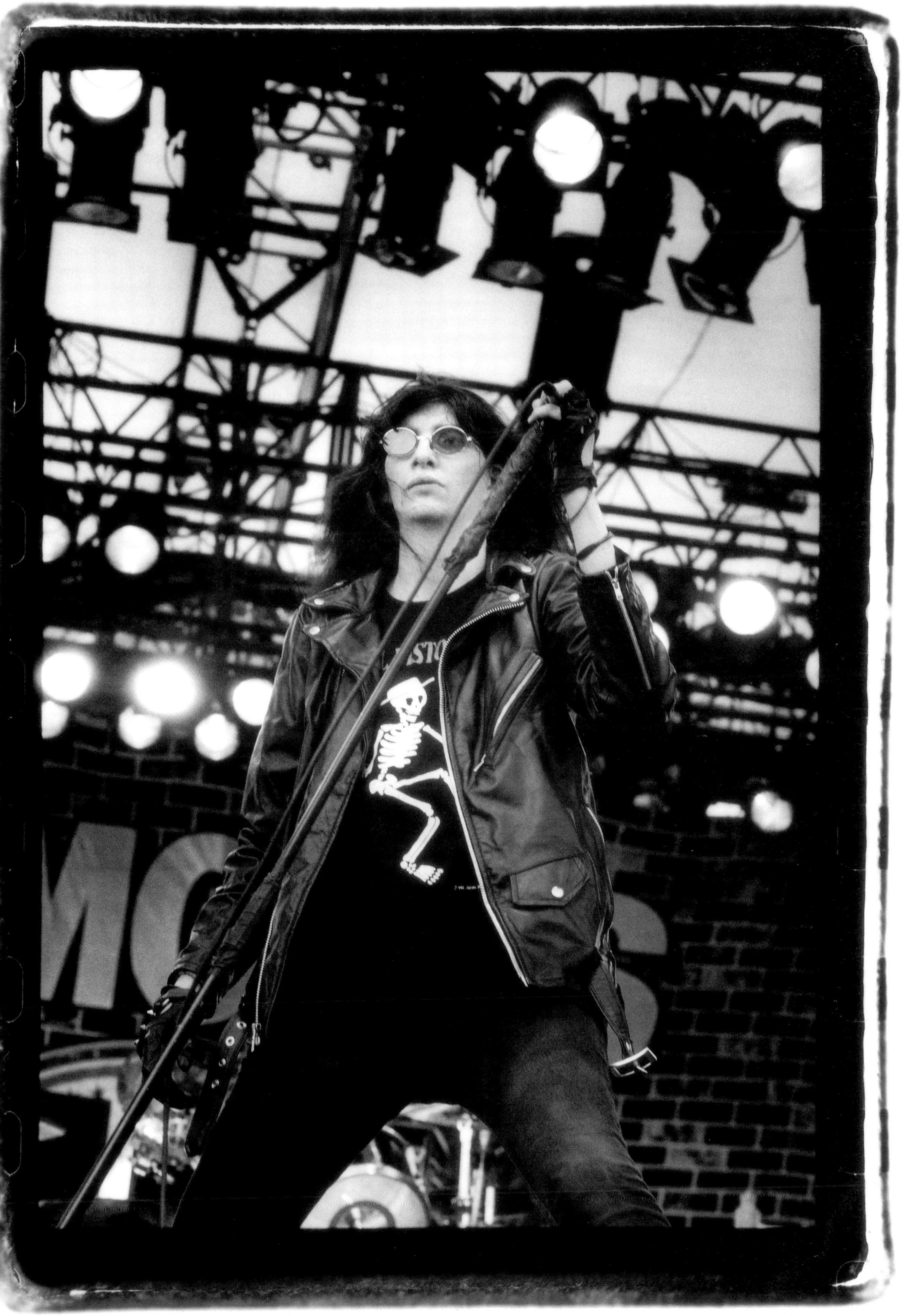

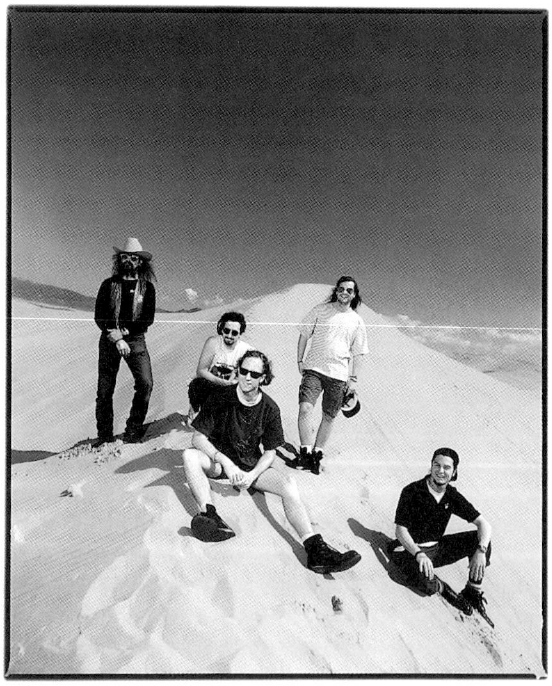

Faith No More
Kelso Dunes

Faith No More
"Corcovado"
Rio

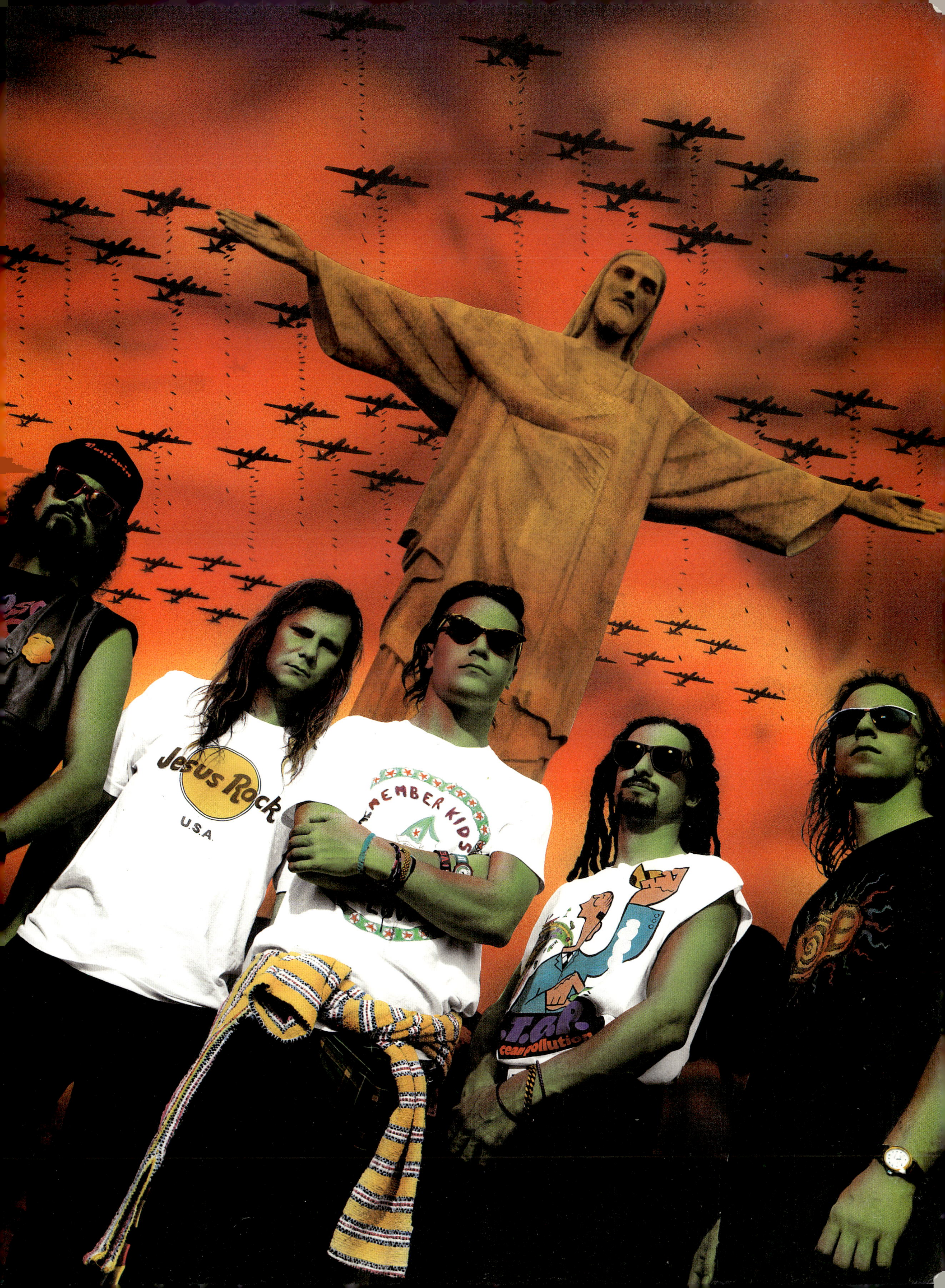
Jesus Rock
U.S.A.
MEMBER KIDS

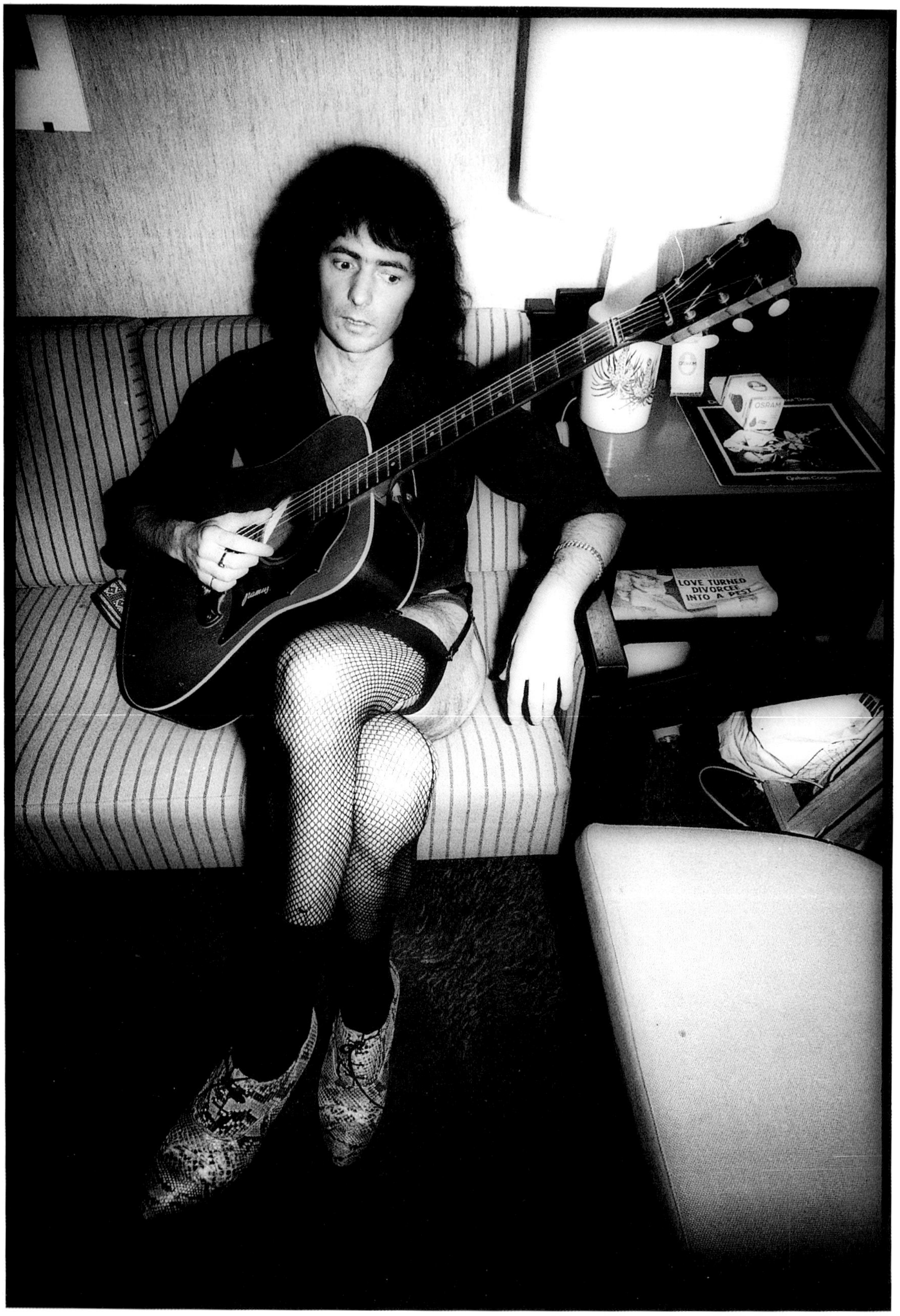

Mr. Blackmore Comes Out
Denmark, '93

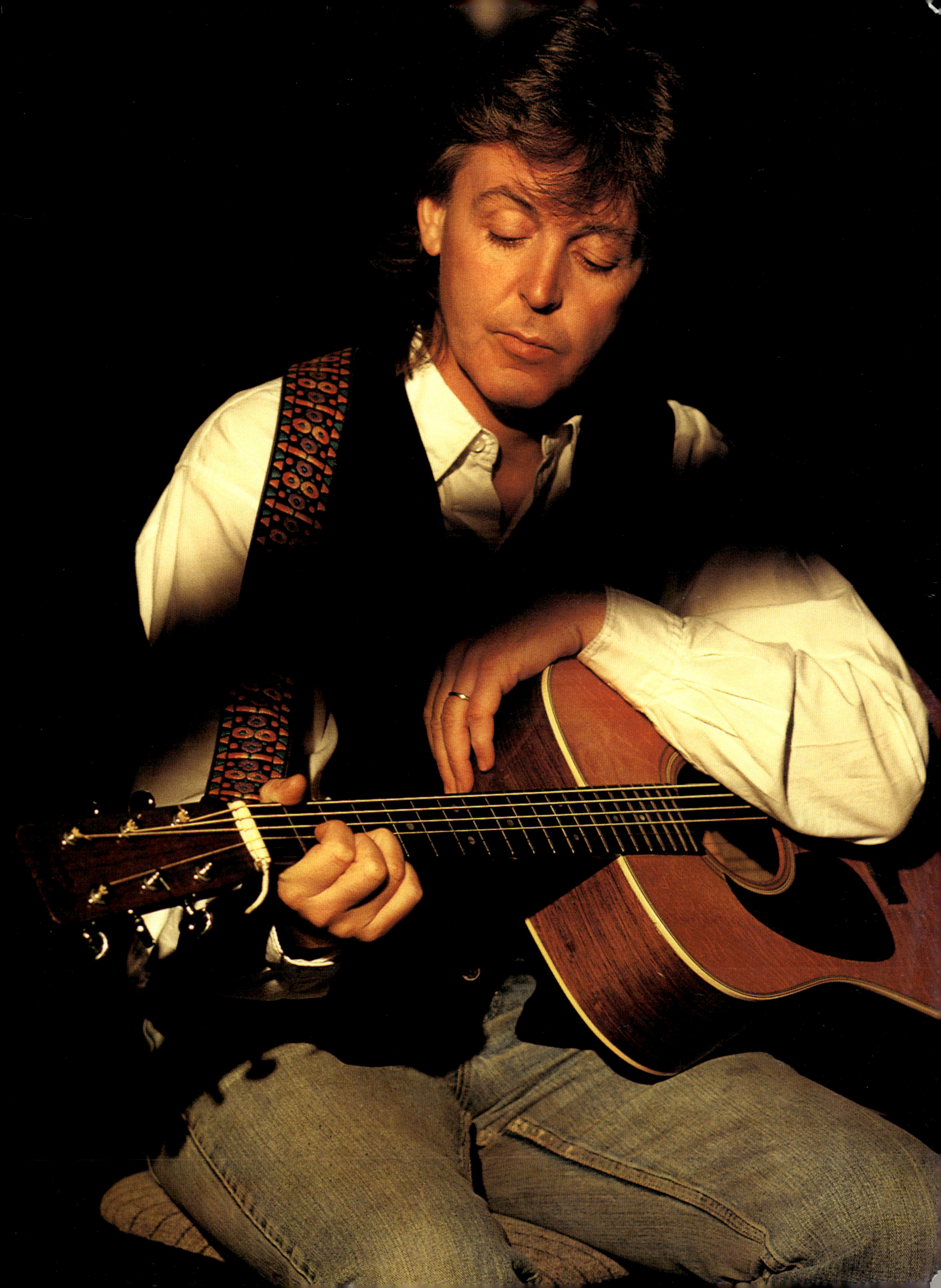

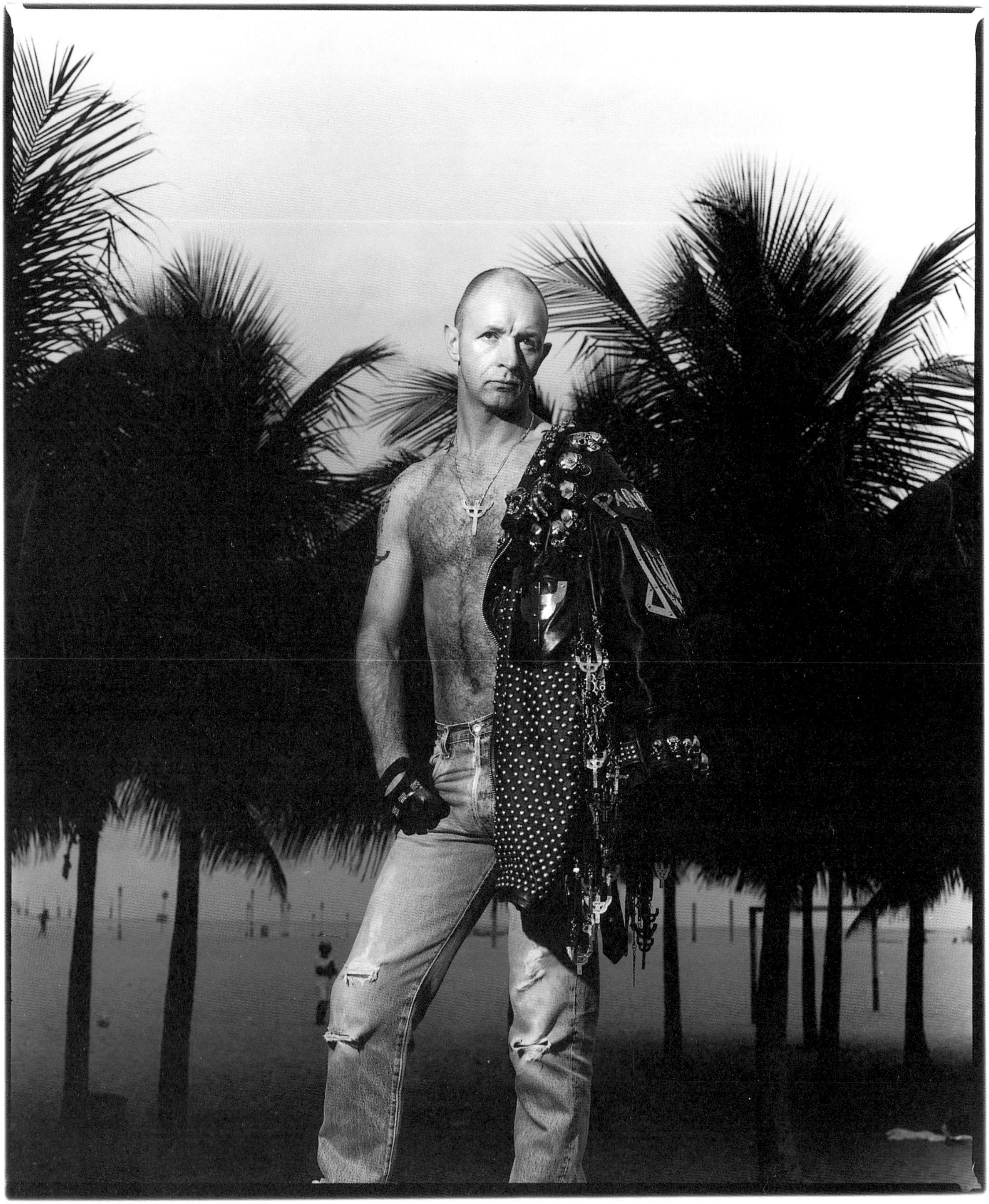

ROB.....

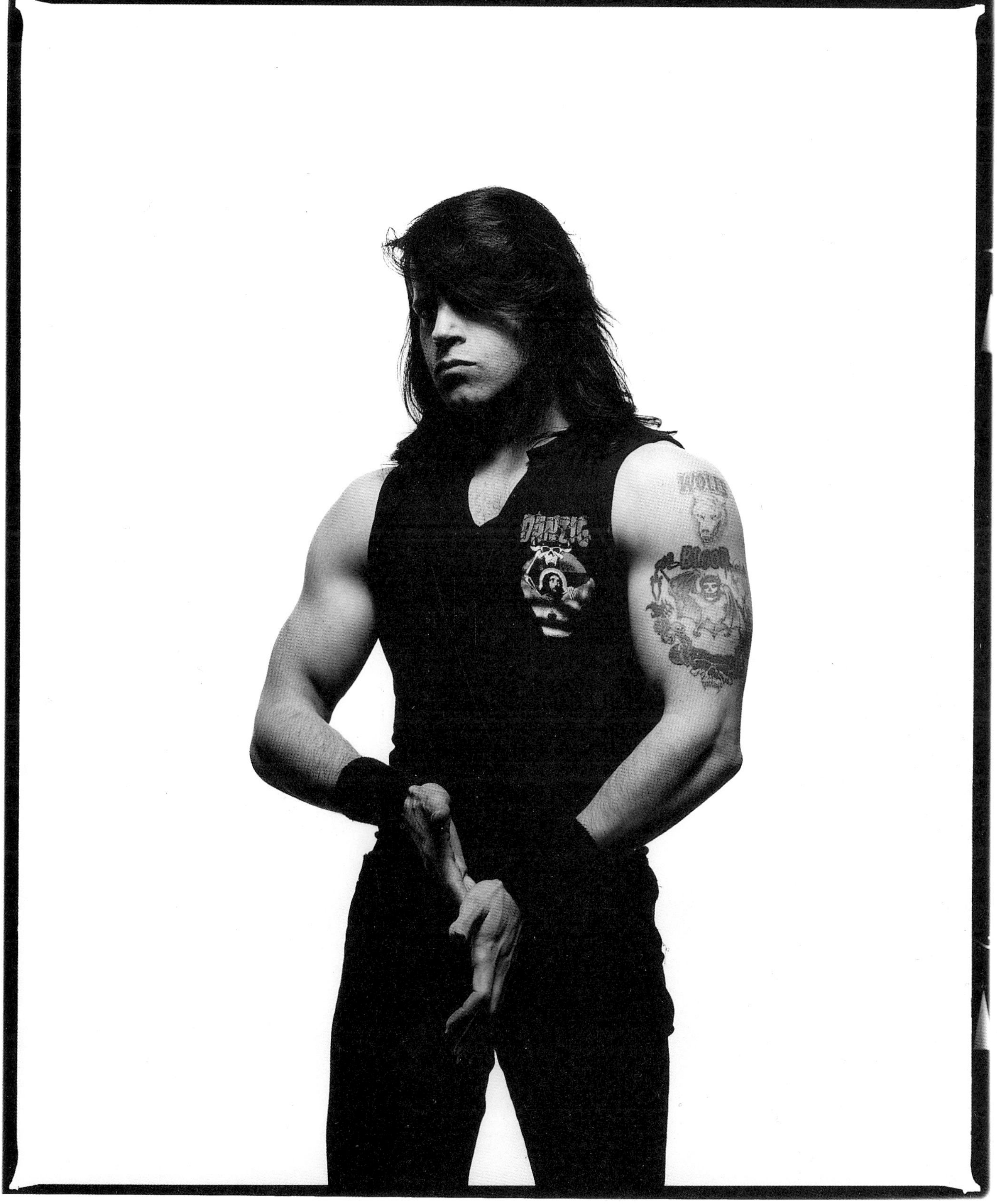

GLENN

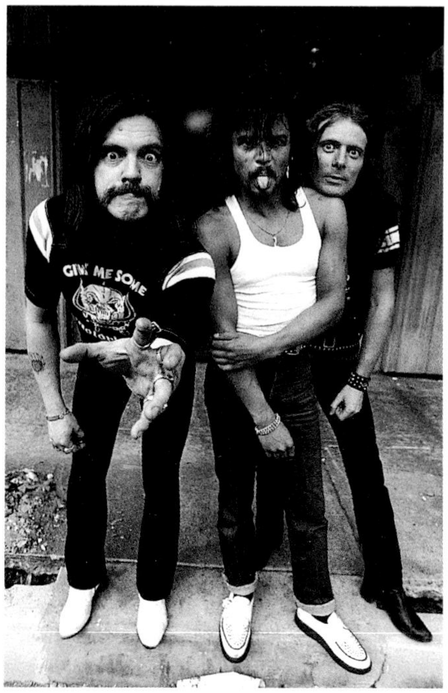

MOTORHEAD
OLD WALDORF, SAN FRANCISCO

LEMMY

Motorhead played the Zeppelin field in Nuremberg. They were opening on a festival. Lemmy walked out and said, "Here's something you fuckers haven't heard for 36 years" and let off an air raid siren. And the band went right into their song "Bomber." After the song there was silence. He said, "Have you not got a sense of humor?" It was deathly silent.

ROSS HALFIN

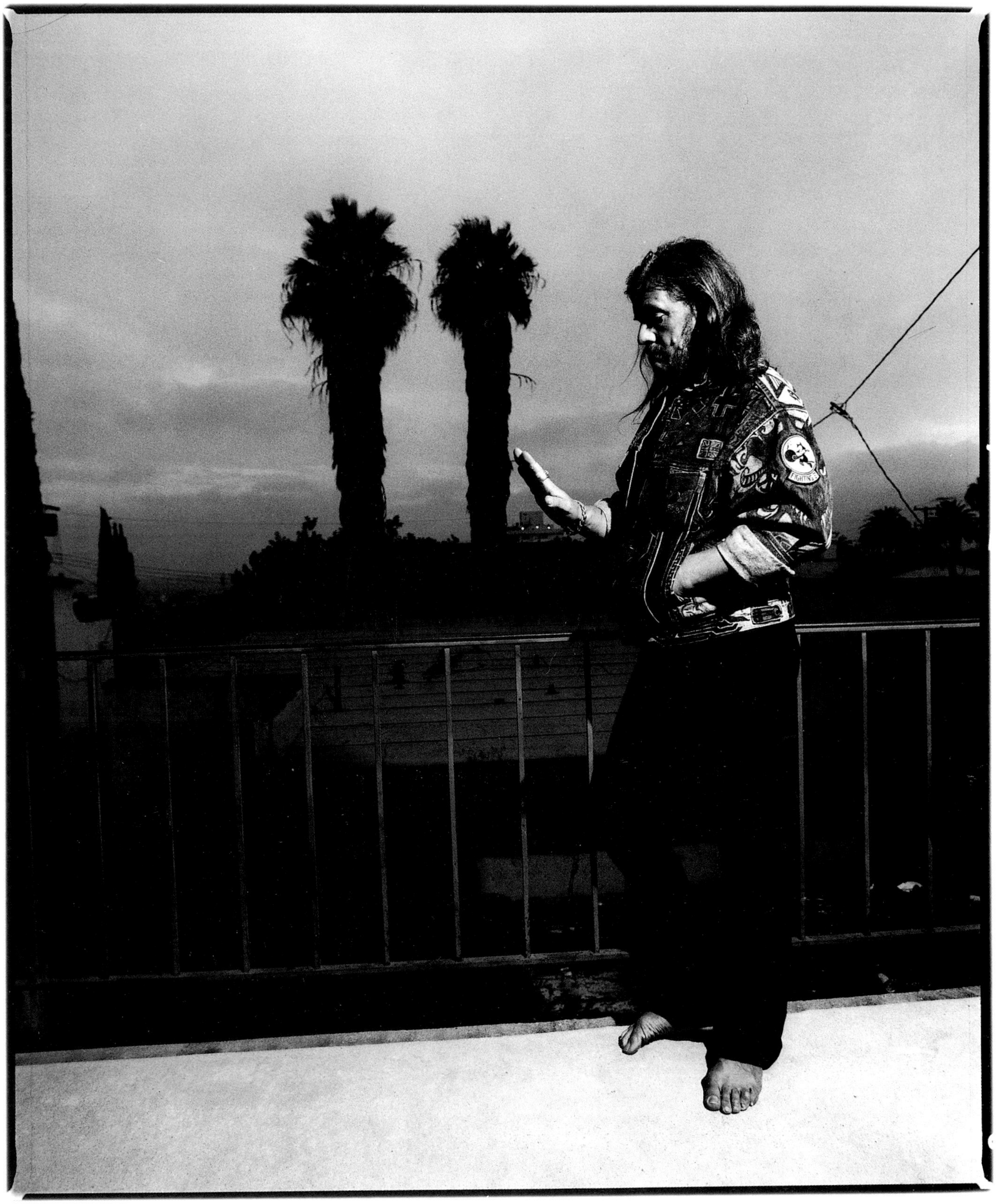

Lemmy
Hollywood, '92

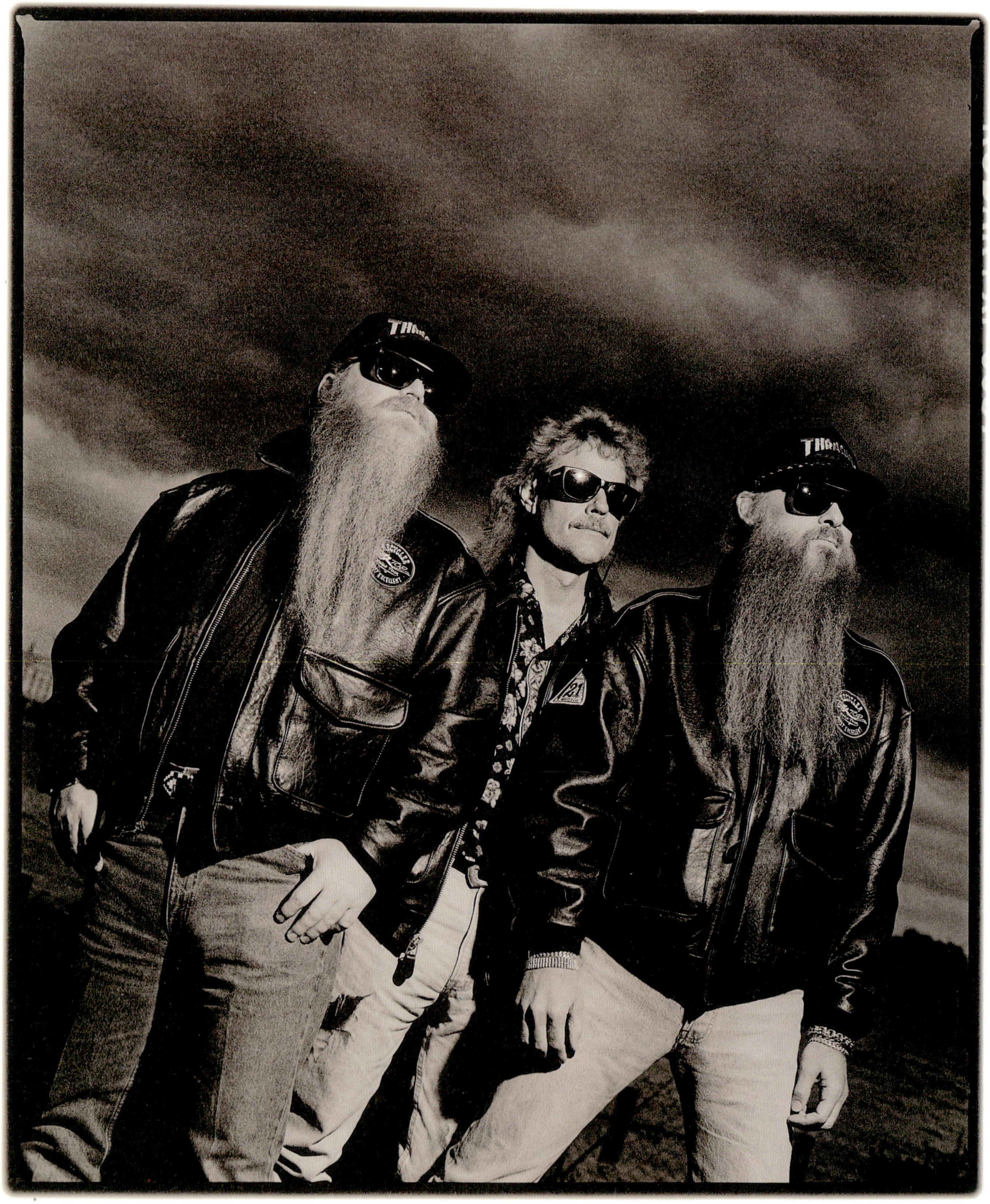

Z Z Top
Hamburg, '91

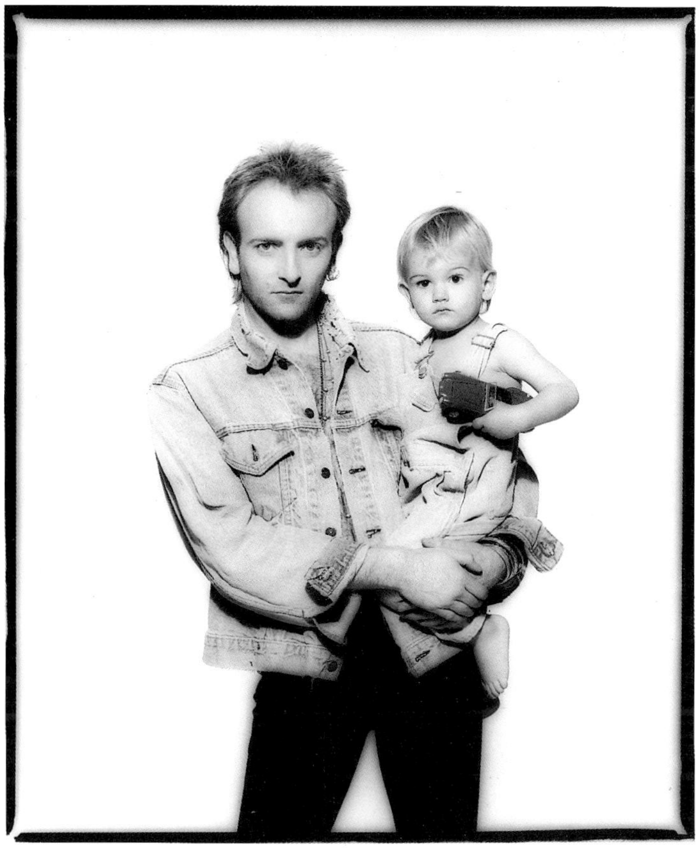

The Boys

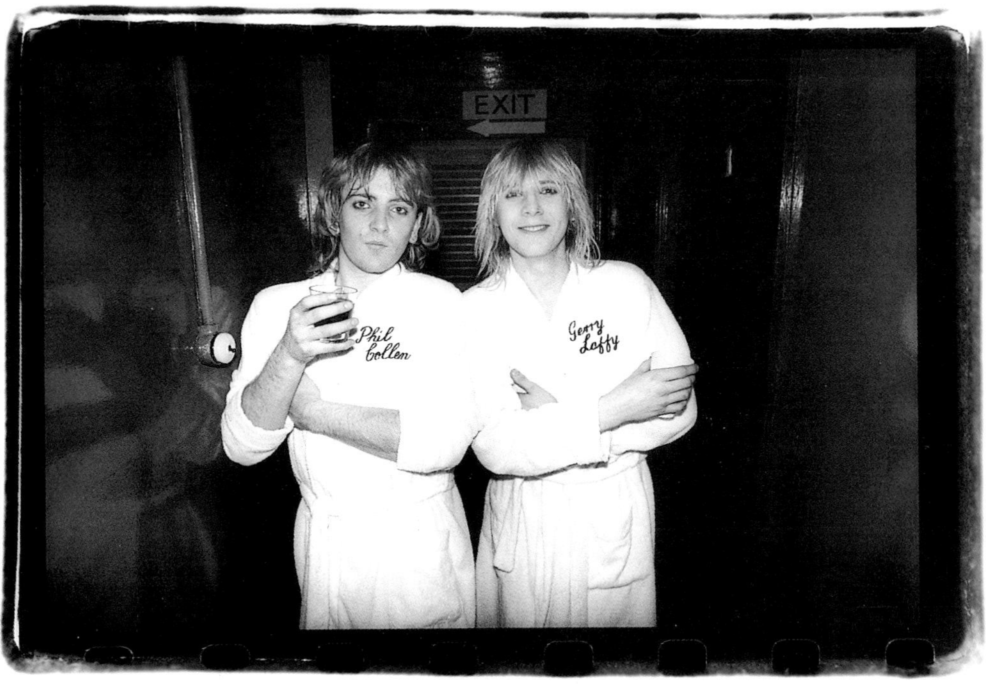

And The Girls

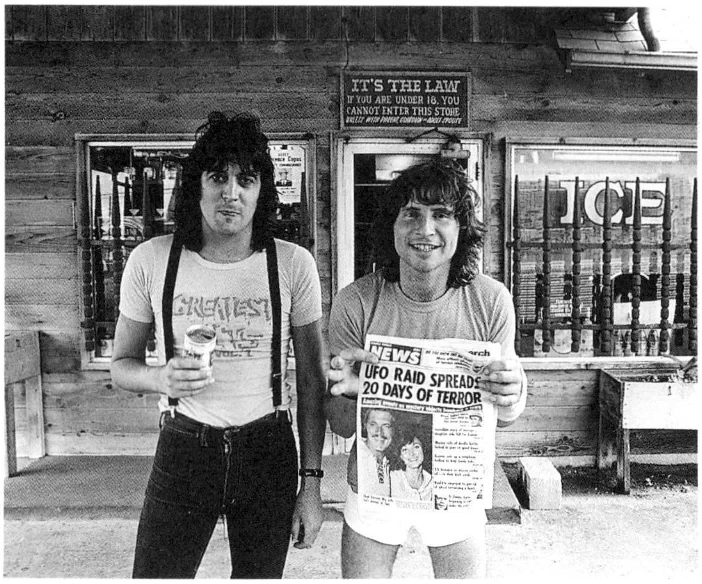
IT'S THE LAW
IF YOU ARE UNDER 16, YOU
CANNOT ENTER THIS STORE
ICE
GREATEST
NEWS
UFO RAID SPREADS
20 DAYS OF TERROR

U.F.O.

"The first band I toured America with"

–Ross Halfin

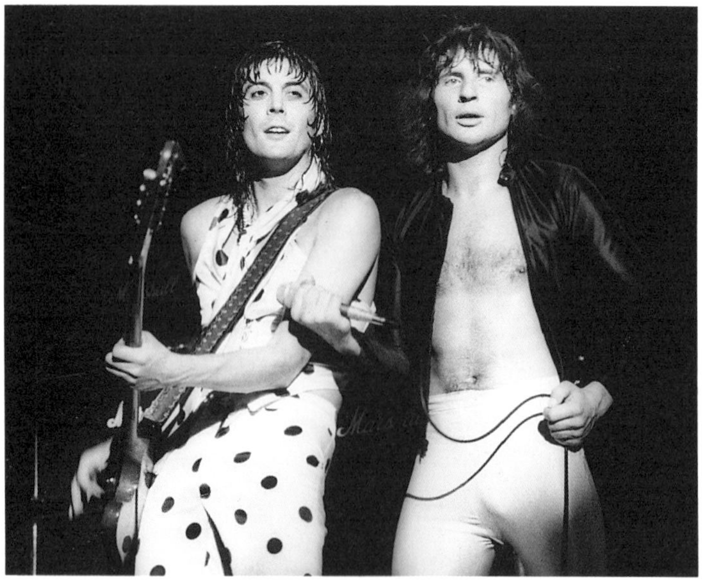

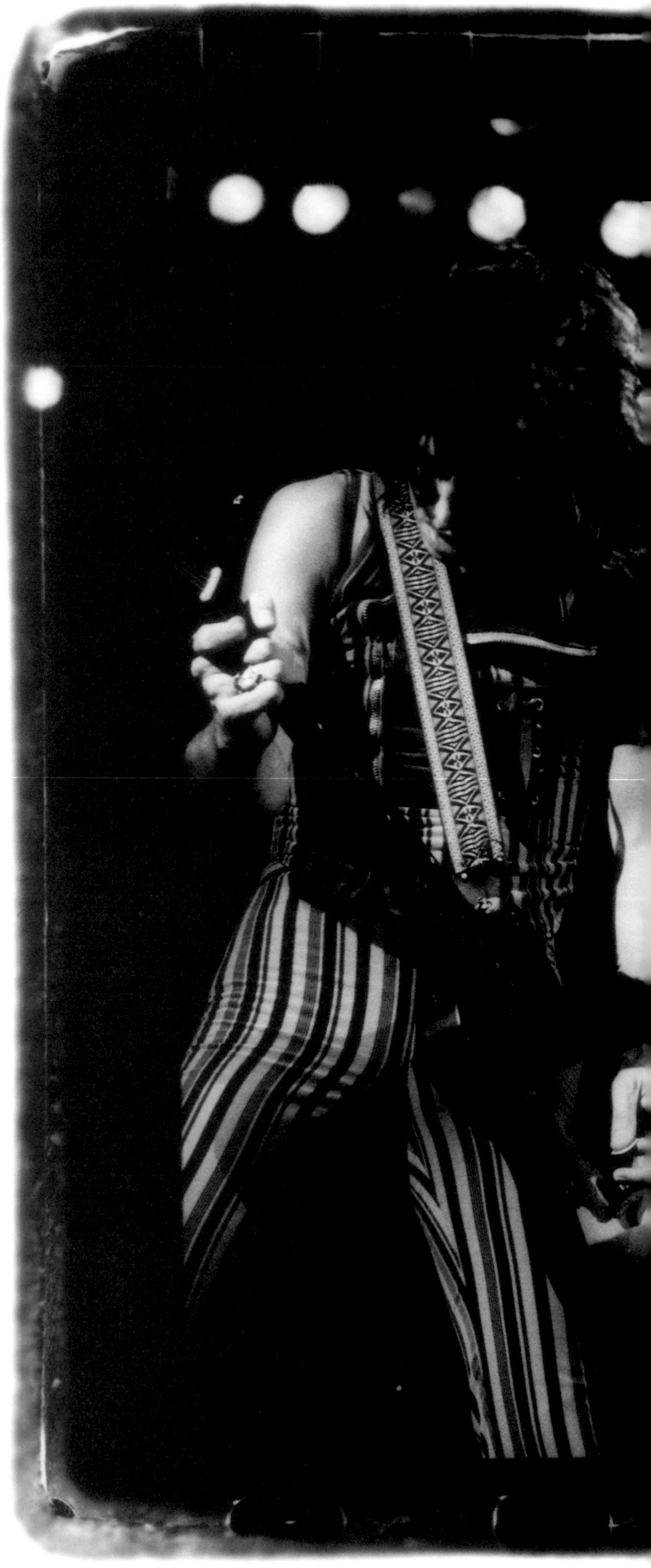

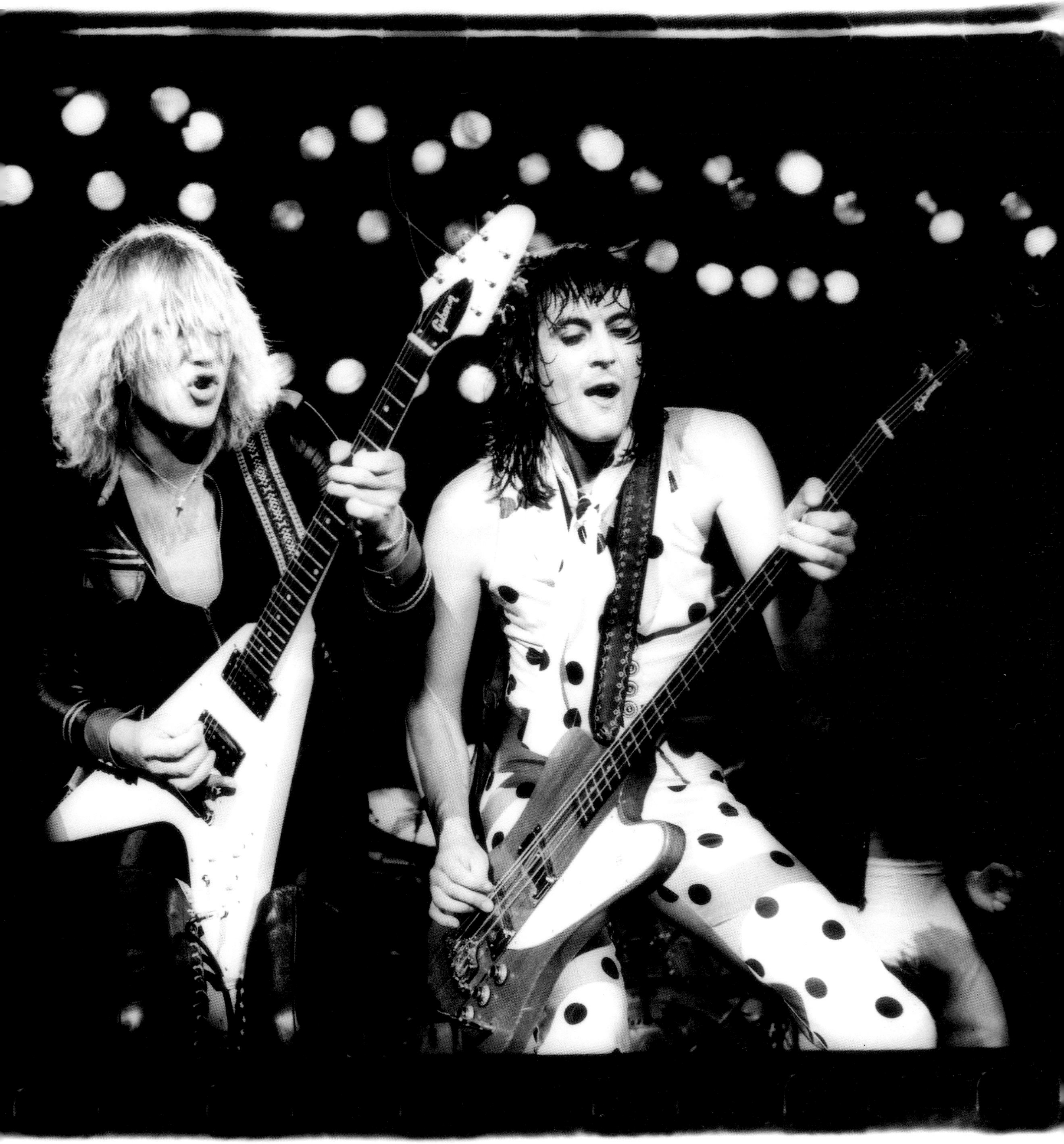

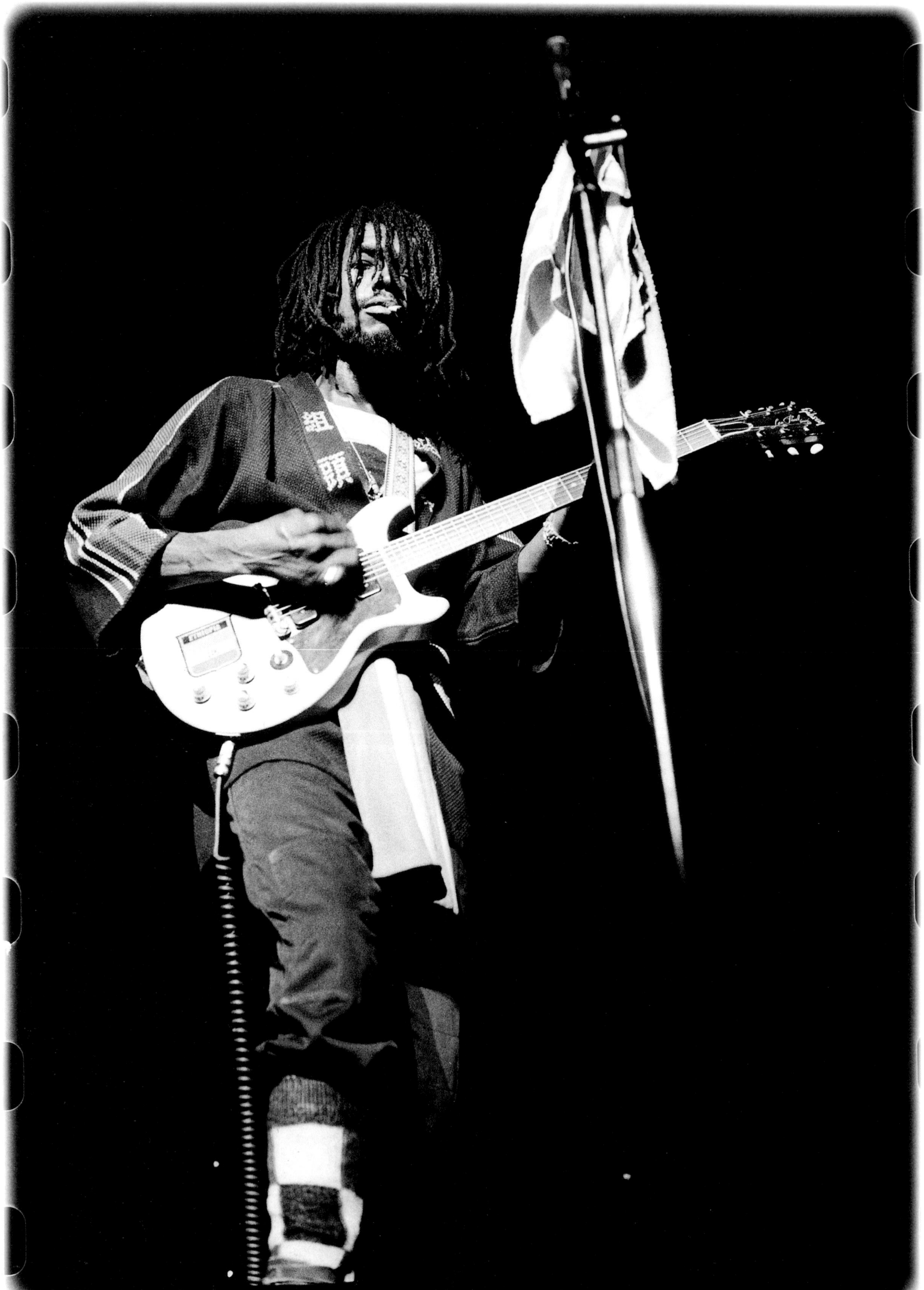

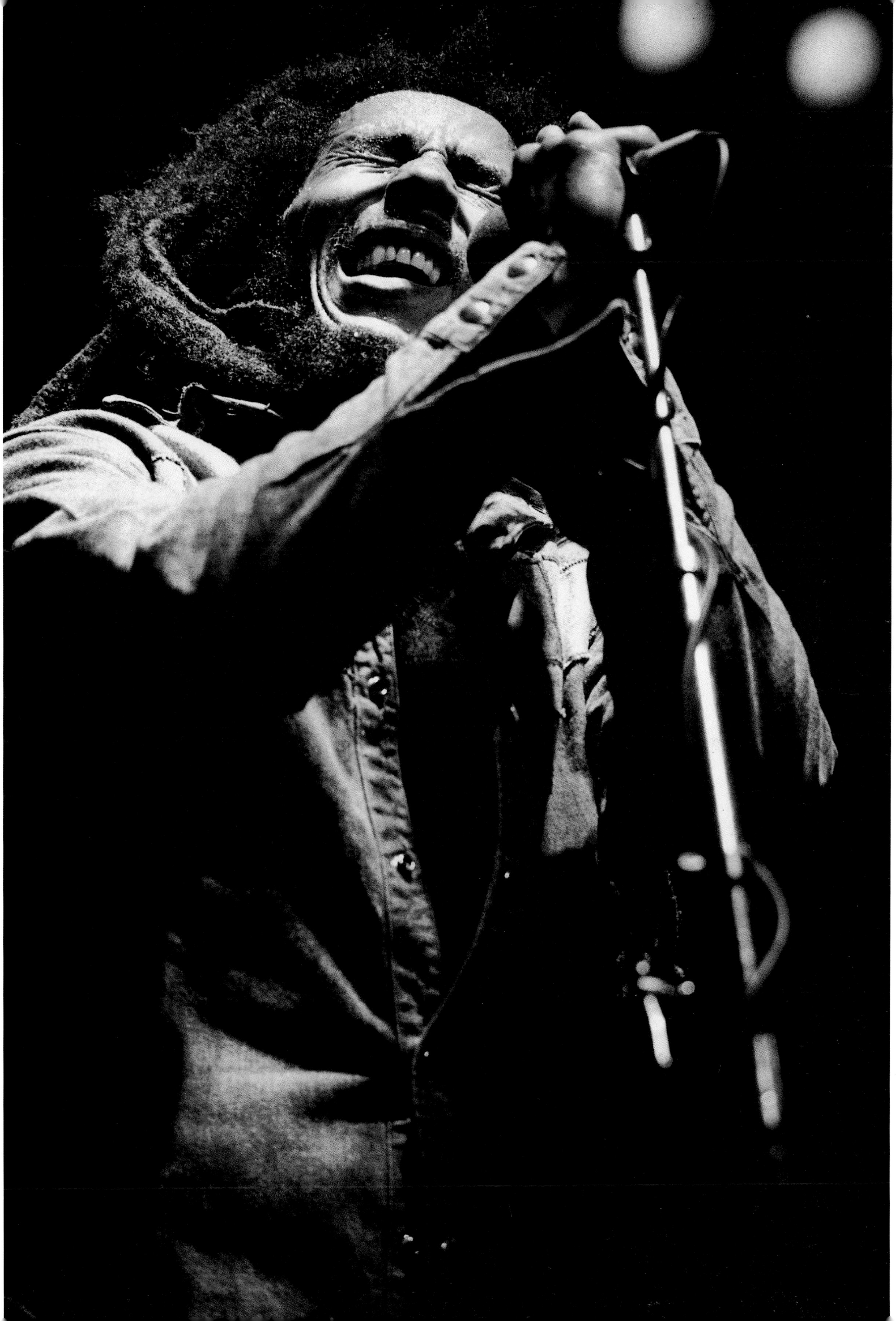

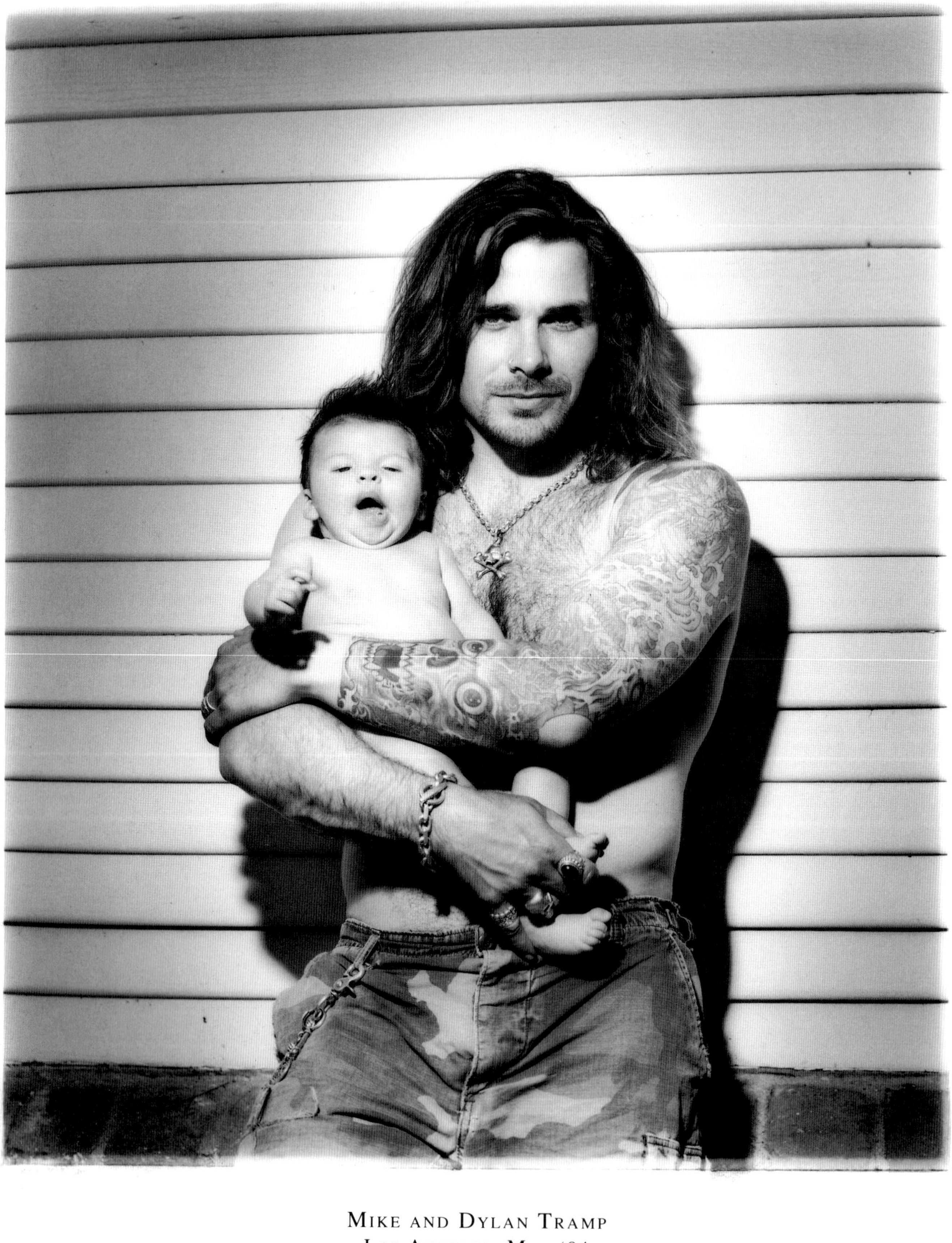

Mike and Dylan Tramp
Los Angeles, May '94

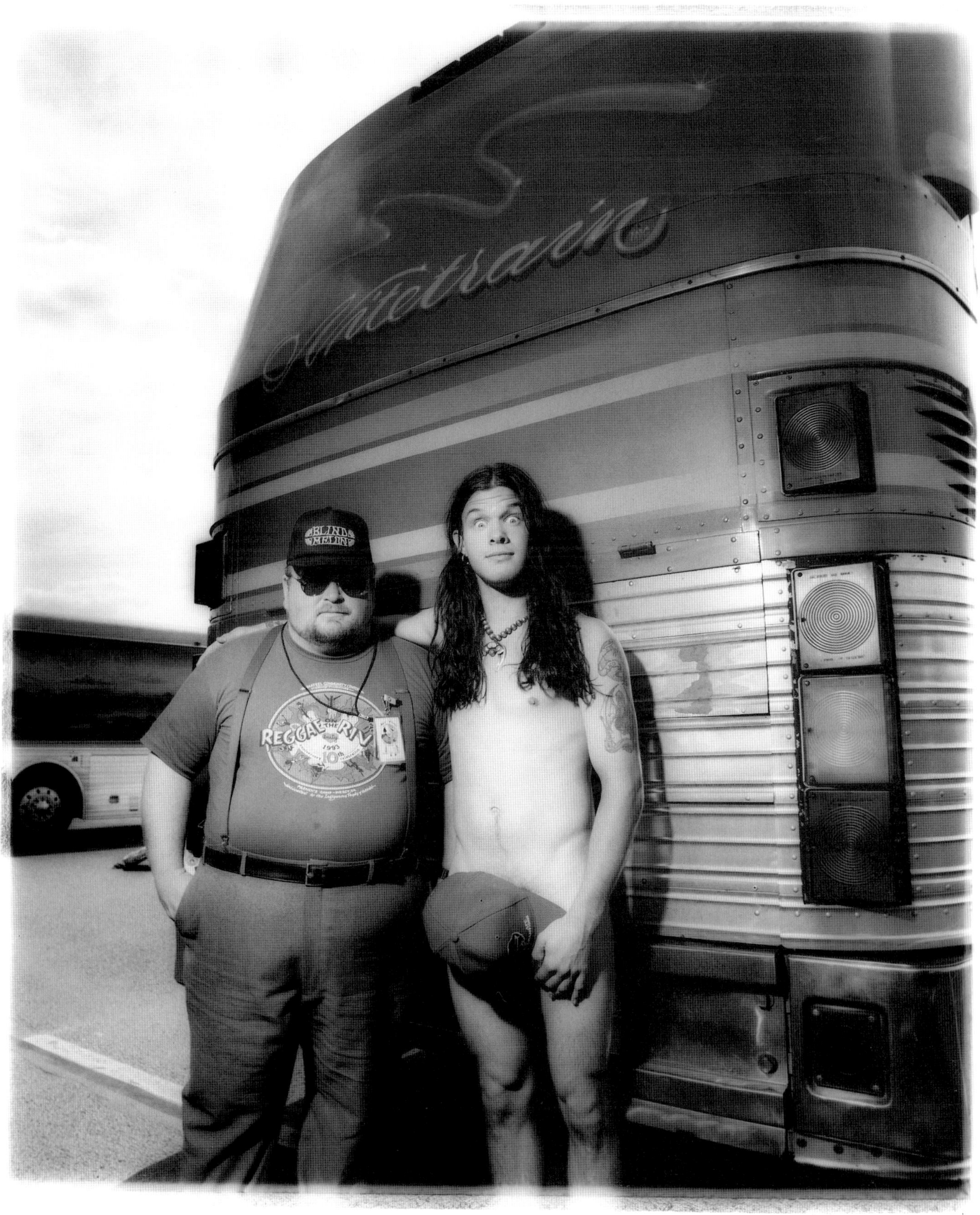

SHANNON HOON AND DRIVER
BOSTON '94

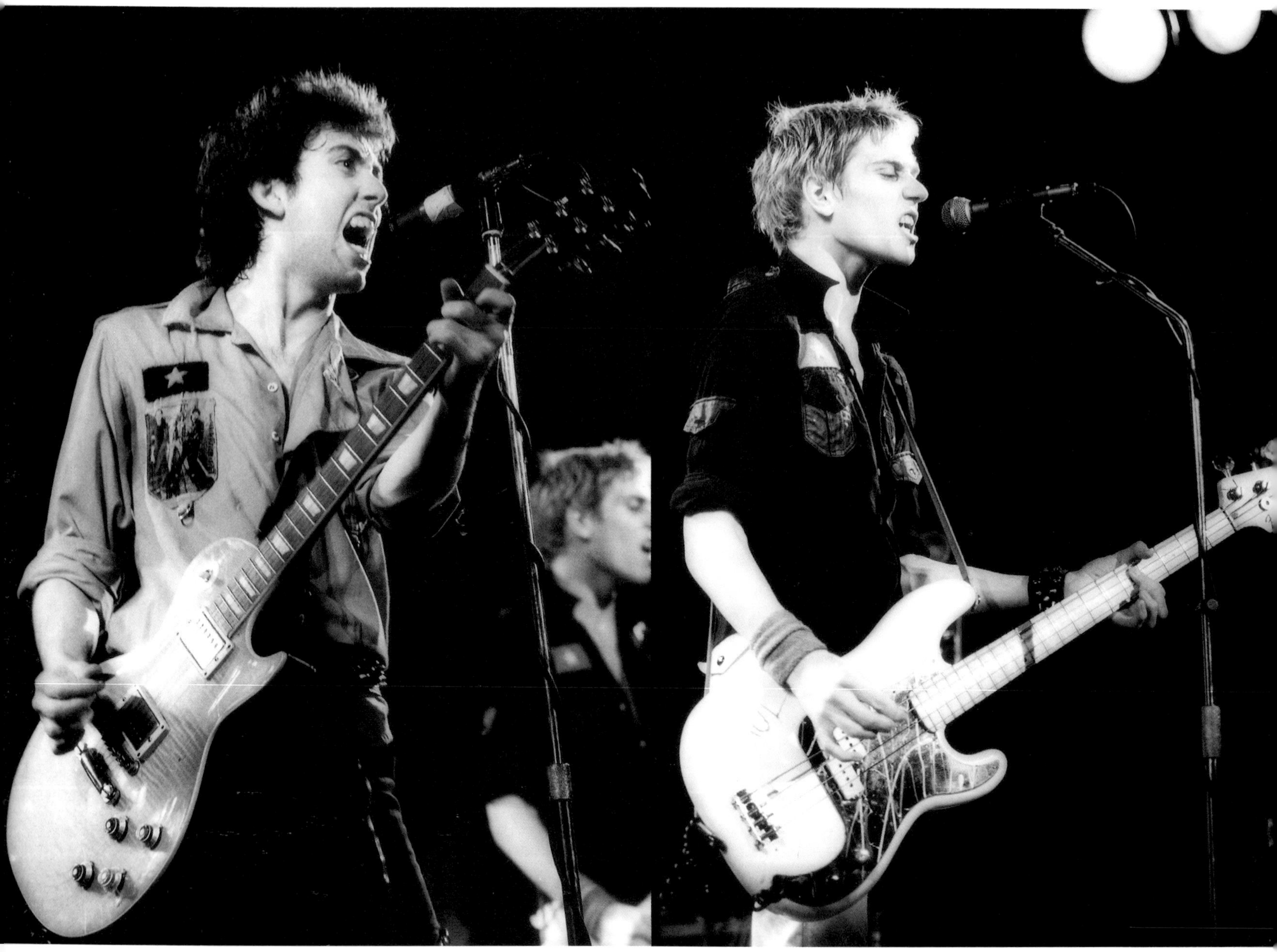

THE CLASH

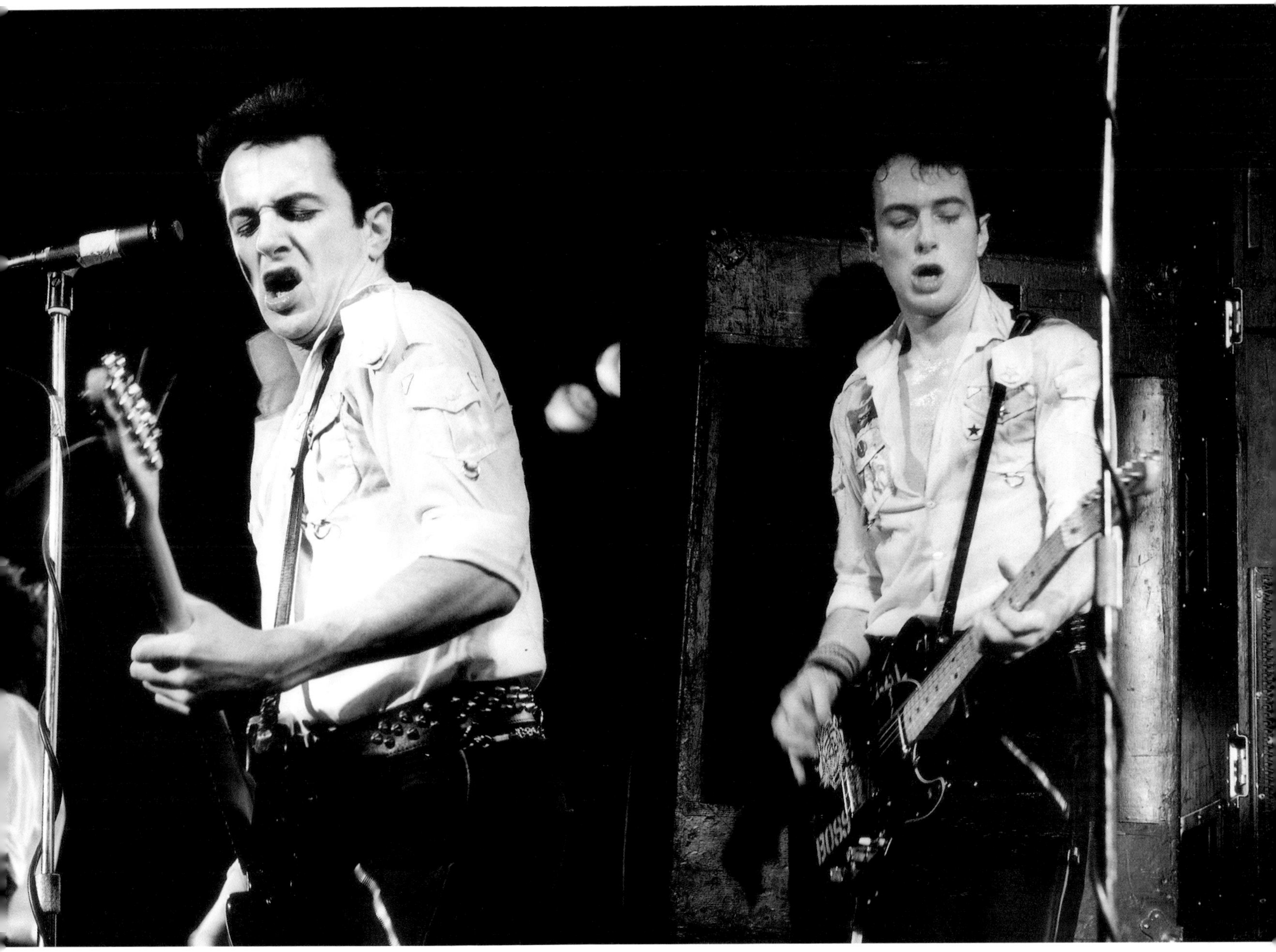
BOSS

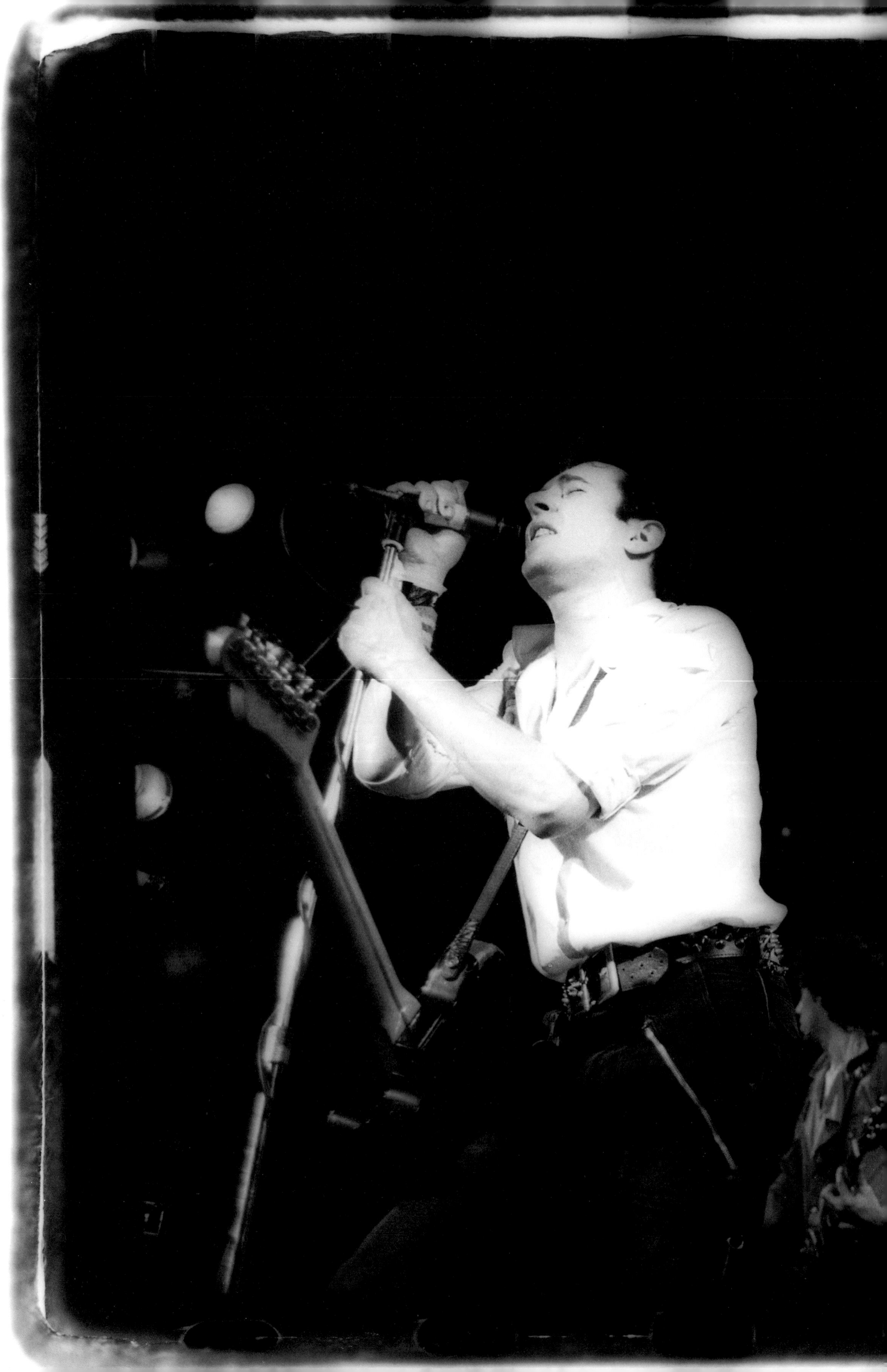

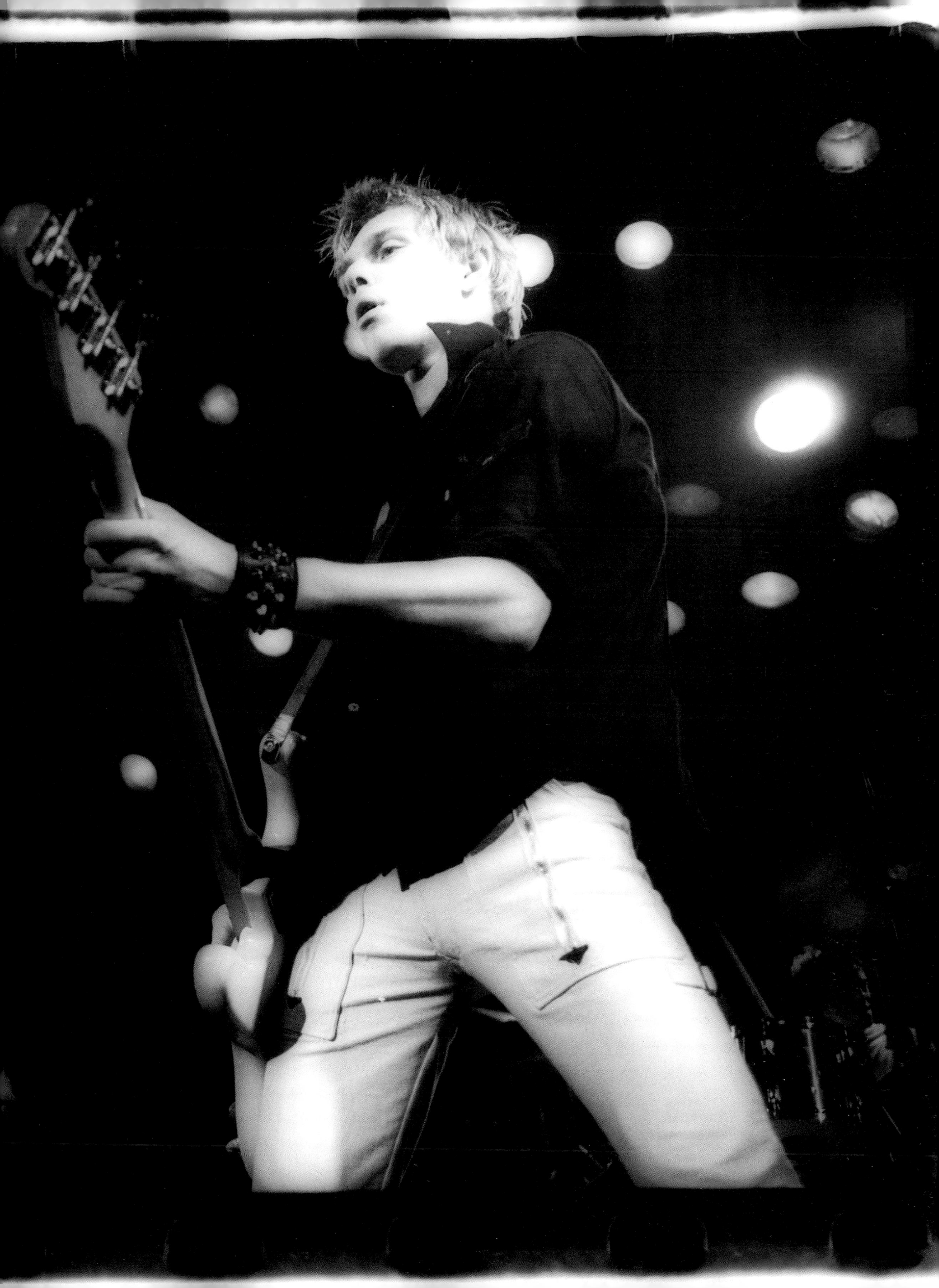

black sabbath

If fuckin' Tchaikovsky got himself out of the grave and fuckin' came on and did the most fantastic fuckin' concert in the world - they'd turn around and say, "Shit!"

Sabbath Drummer Bill Ward
on the press

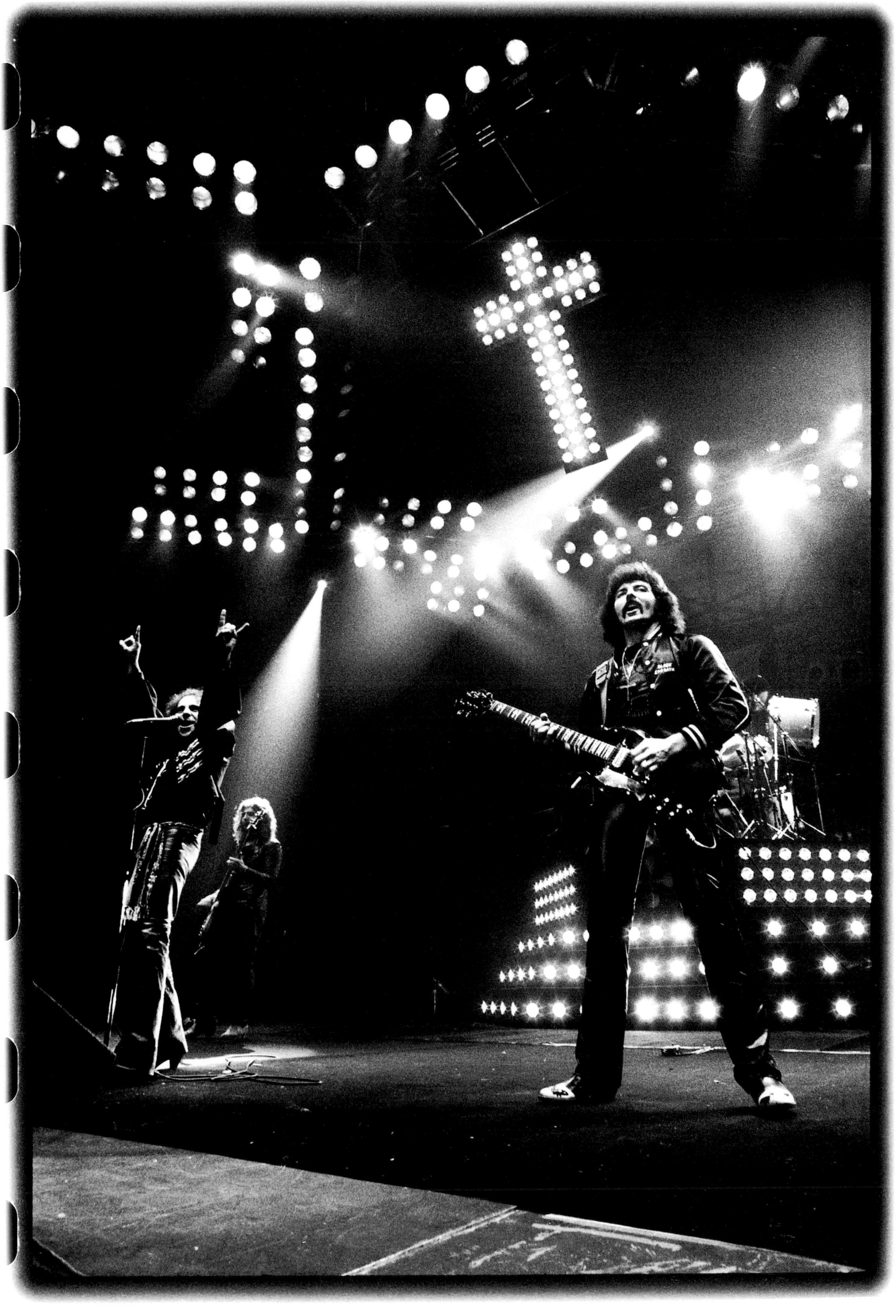

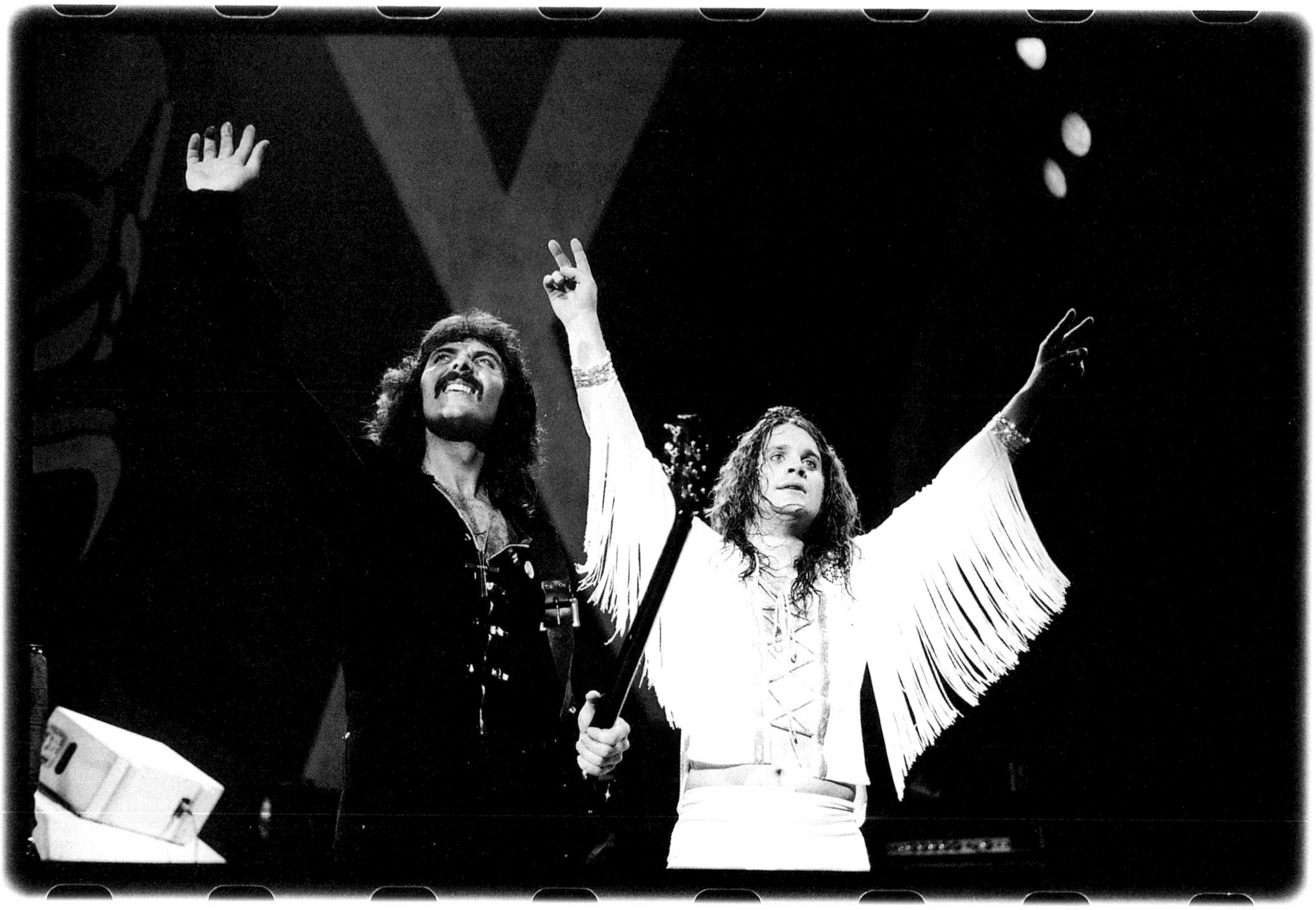

TONY IOMMI AND OZZY OSBOURNE

BLACK SABBATH

Critics said they couldn't play. Critics are people who make their living writing about themselves listening to records – so fuck them. Truth is, Geezer Butler and Bill Ward are one of the best rhythm sections that ever existed. The singer wasn't a sex symbol. Songs about smacked out Viet Nam vets. Nuclear devastation, alienation, revenge and other things that make you feel at home with your displacement. And then there was that sound... Thick and malevolent. Ugly and powerful like a heavy blunt instrument held by someone who had about enough. Genius in its feral, slow walking fury. Sabbath was what all the scary guys who stood outside house parties drinking beers in the cold listened to. Either you get it or you don't. They still matter because bands are still trying to rip off a piece of their world. Wouldn't it be great to make one of those heavy metal bands of today play on the same bill with Sabbath on the Vol. 4 tour? It would be like Godzilla stepping on a cop.

HENRY ROLLINS

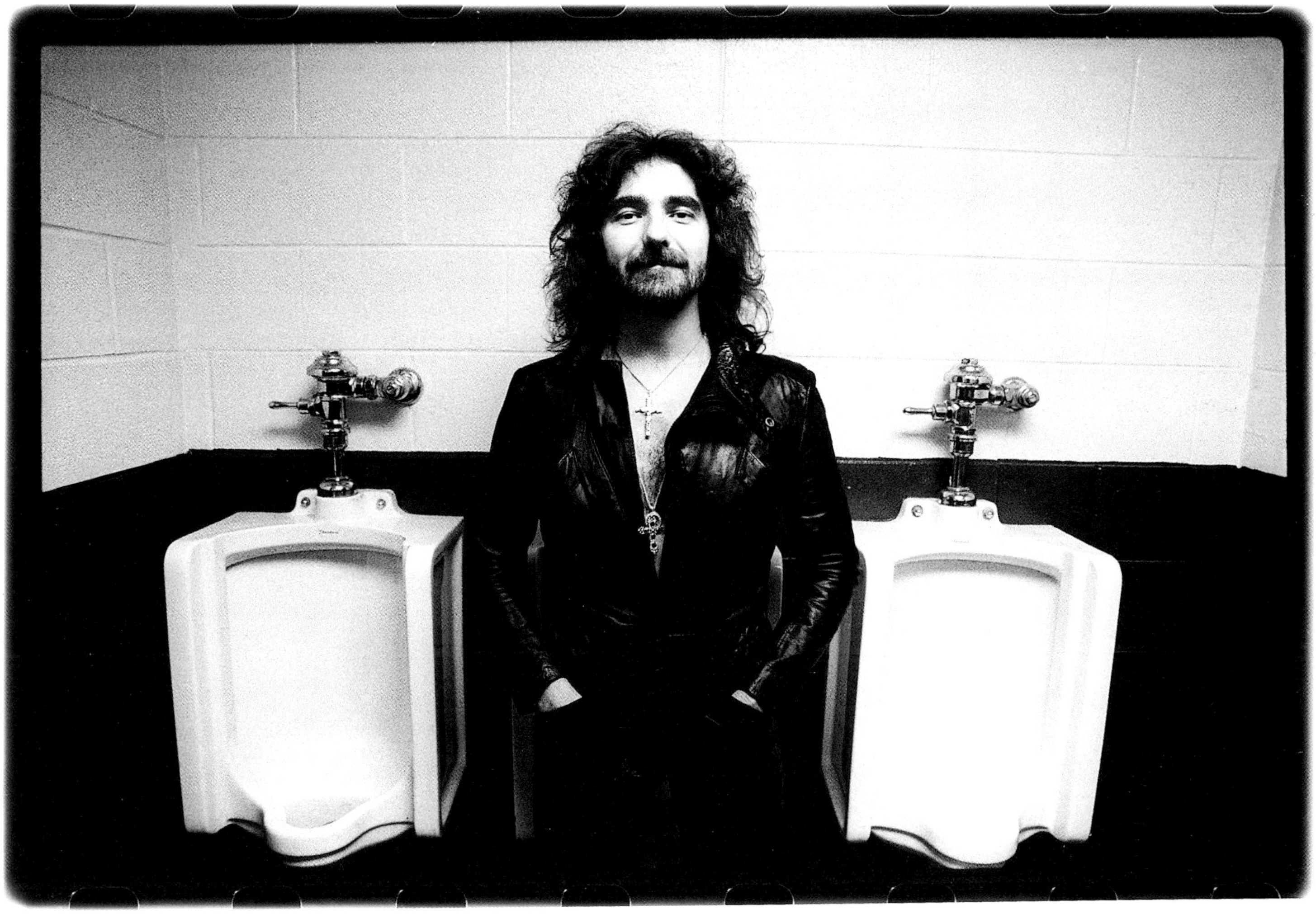

Geezer Butler

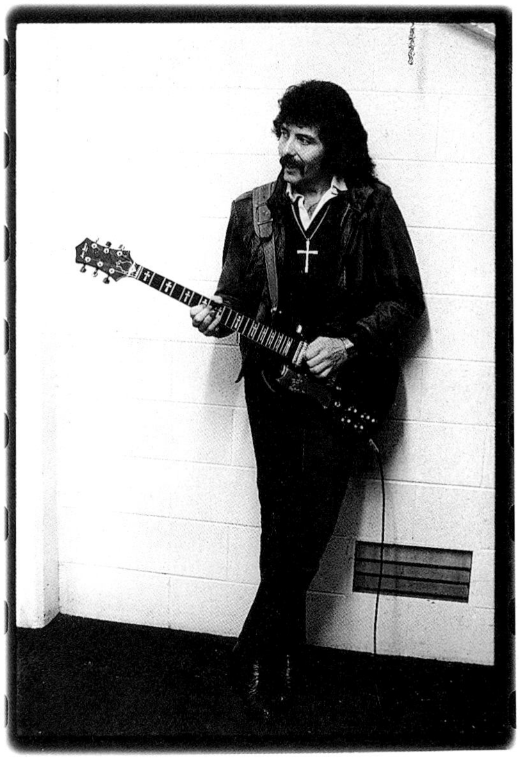

Tony Iommi

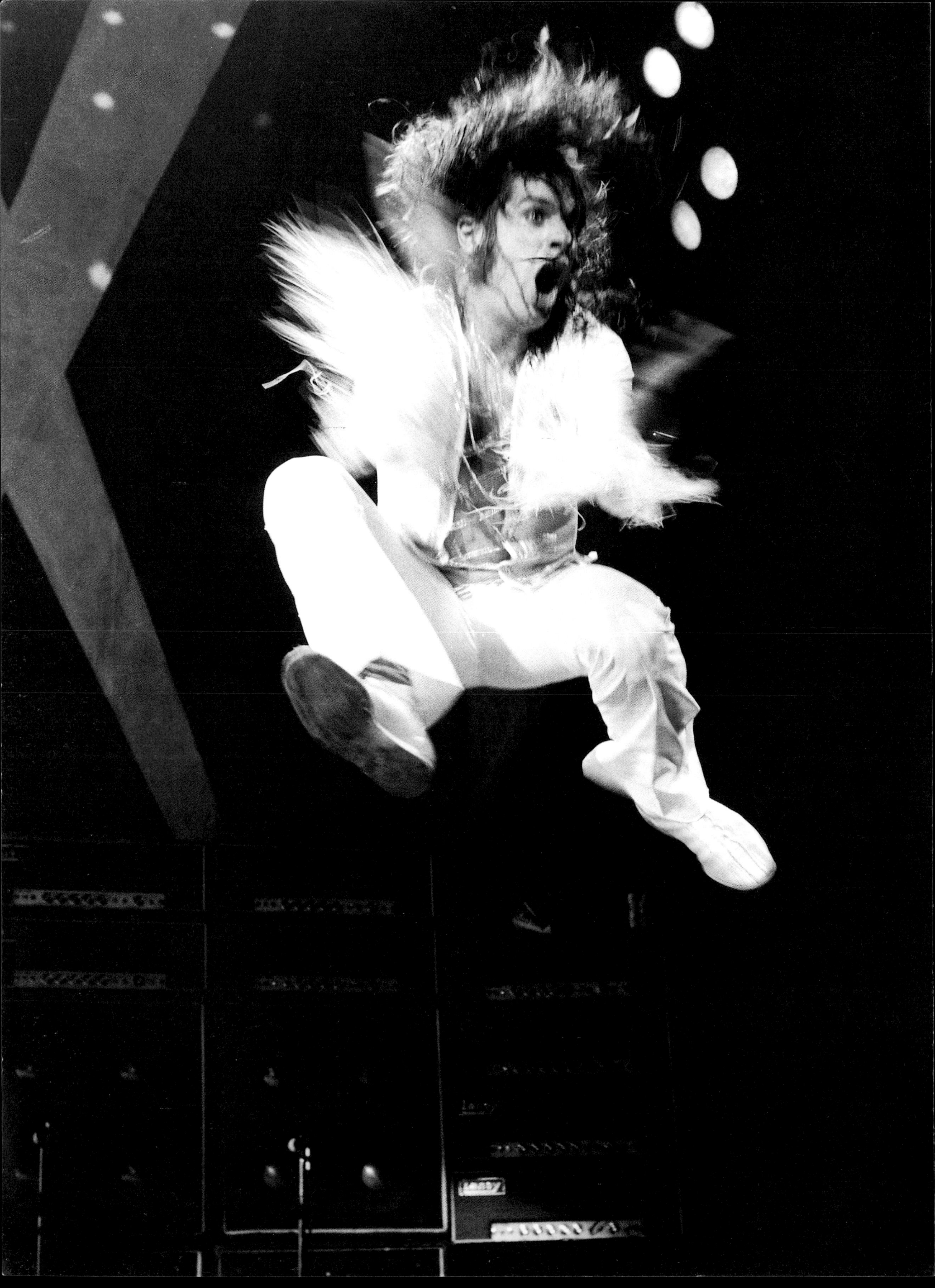

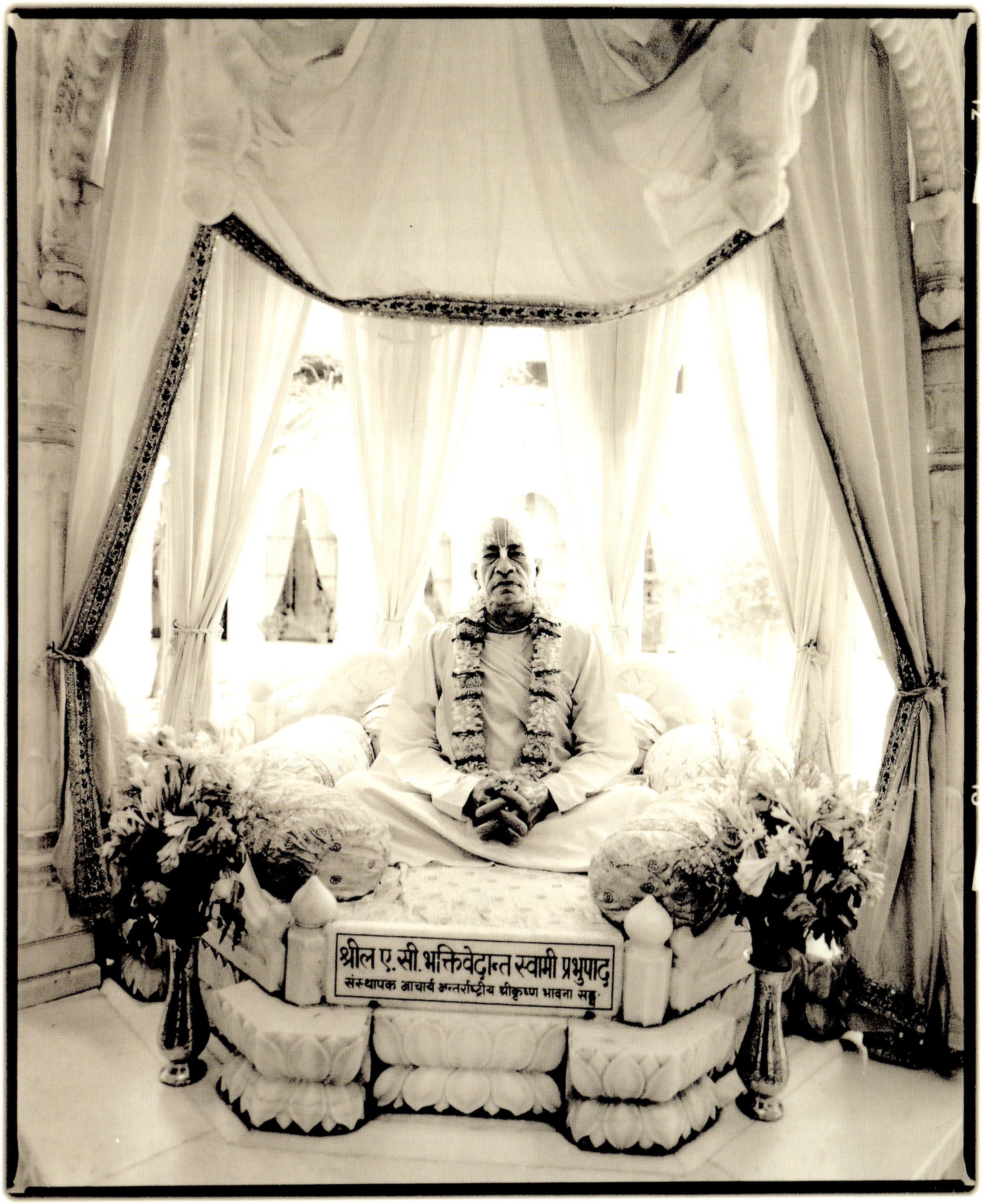

A.C. Bhaktivedanta
Swami Prabhupāda
Bombay, India

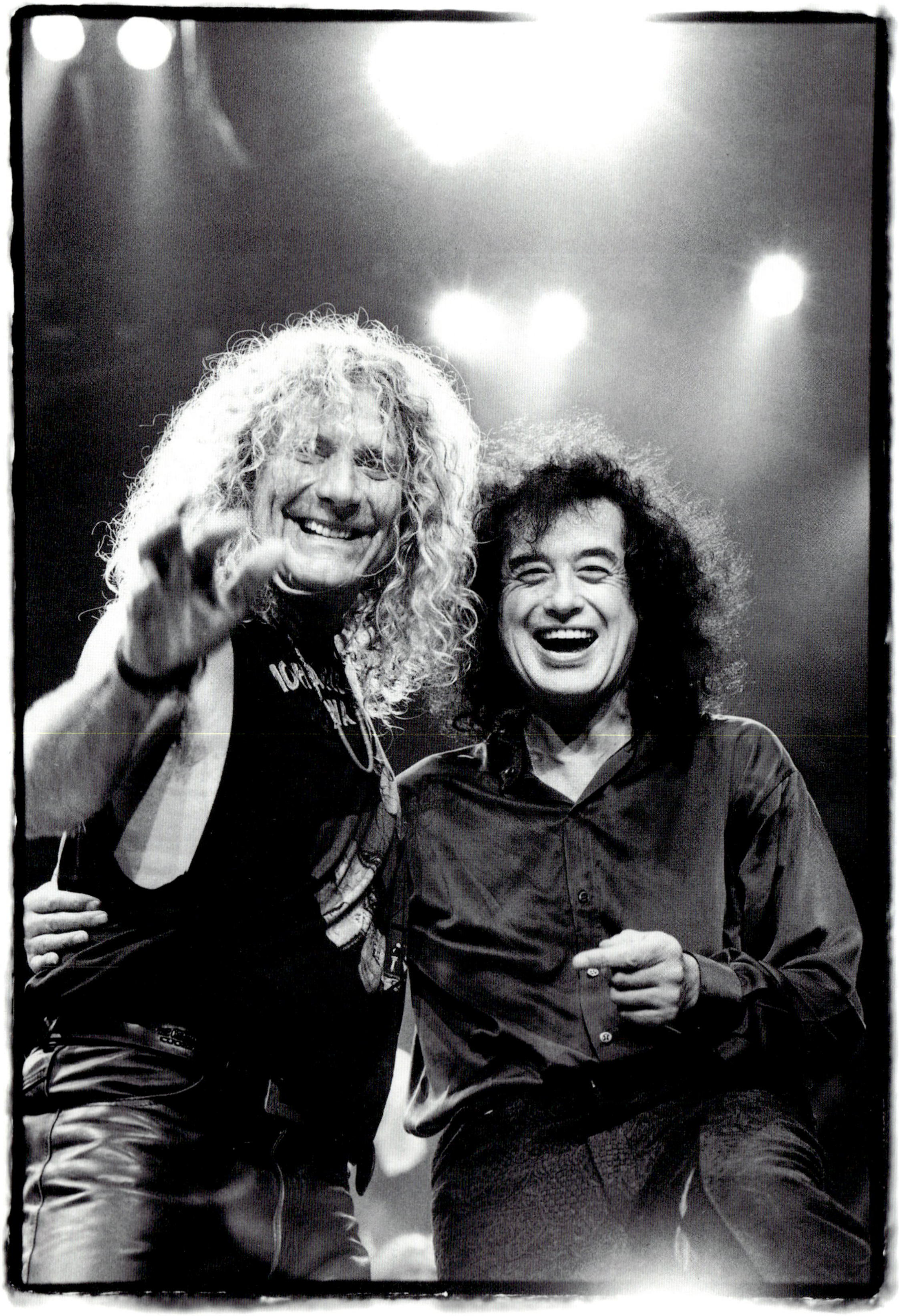

Plant/Page
Flinders Park
Melbourne, March '96

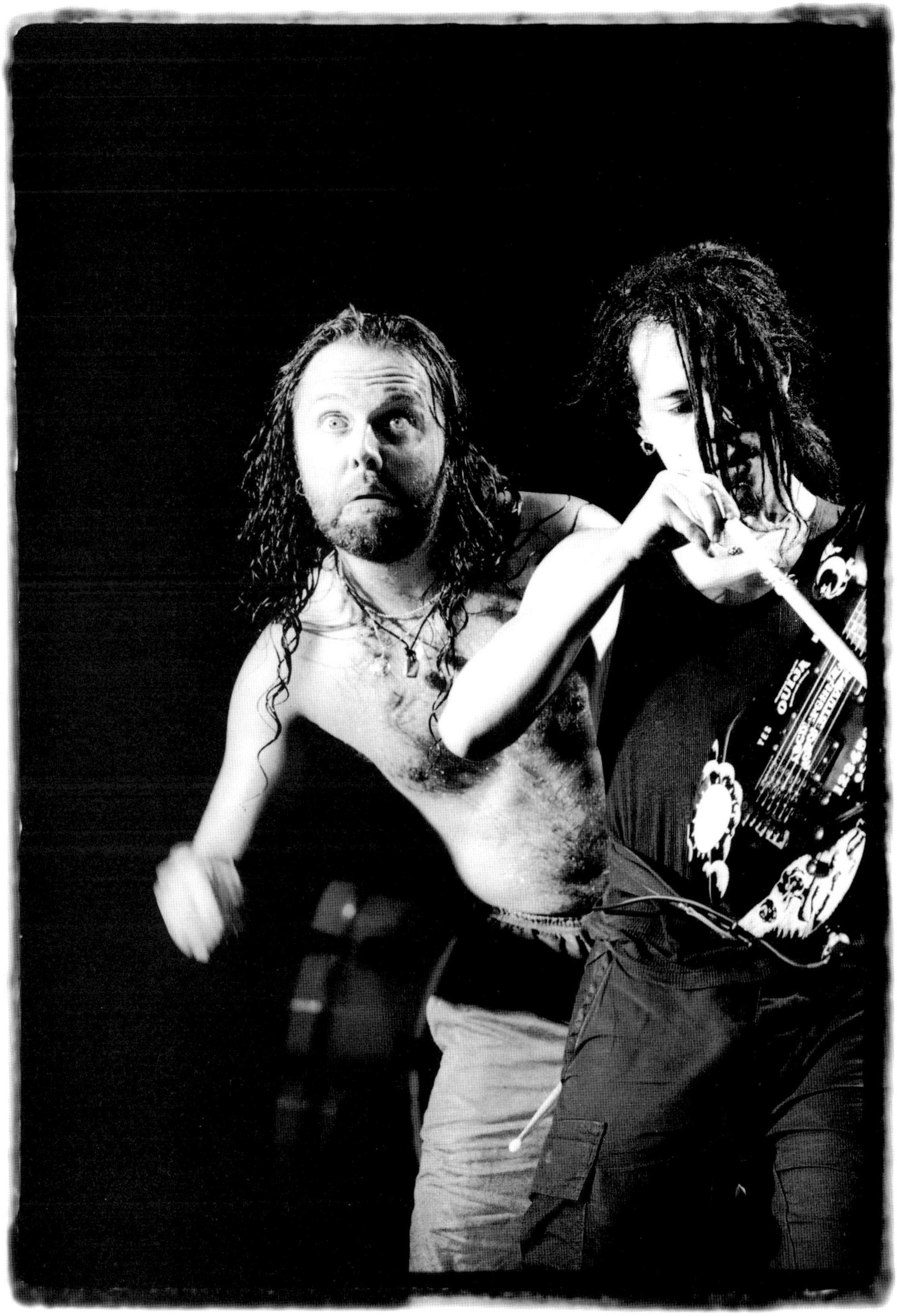

Lars and Kirk
Miami, '94

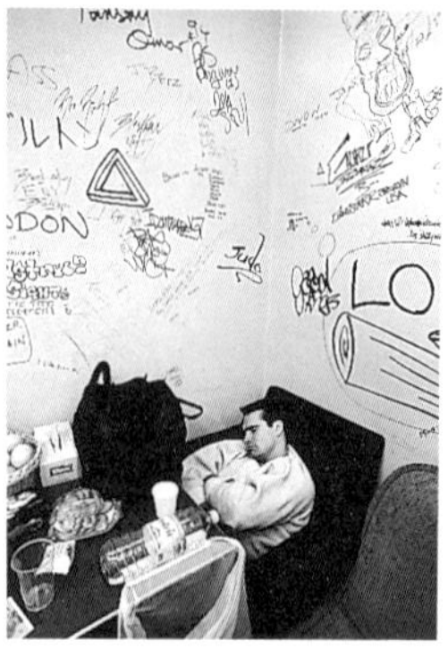

HENRY ROLLINS

Sometimes Hank and I will be onstage and make eye contact and just scream at each other out of sheer joy. Like we're saying, "Let's play so hard that we just explode, OK?"

One time we were playing somewhere in upstate New York in a place with just the worst PA. Basically somebody's hi-fi and through the course of the gig, various bits of it were blowing up. Toward the end Hank just put down the mike (which wasn't working anyway) and just did his vocals without it. And you could hear him. It was one of the most amazing moments we've ever had. Sheer will. The audience was in a kind of bludgeoned shock. All except one woman on the side of the stage going, "Search And Destroy.....Yee-hah!" Which was weird. It was Tanya Tucker. Things got kind of strange after that.

I think part of the appeal of the Rollins band is people's vicarious pleasure at watching us twist and shriek and flail around and bleed. It's a kind of shamanism-by-proxy. People get a sense of relief that at least somebody's still out there shrieking, flailing, and blooding.

I can't see us as a lounge act.

CHRIS HASKETT

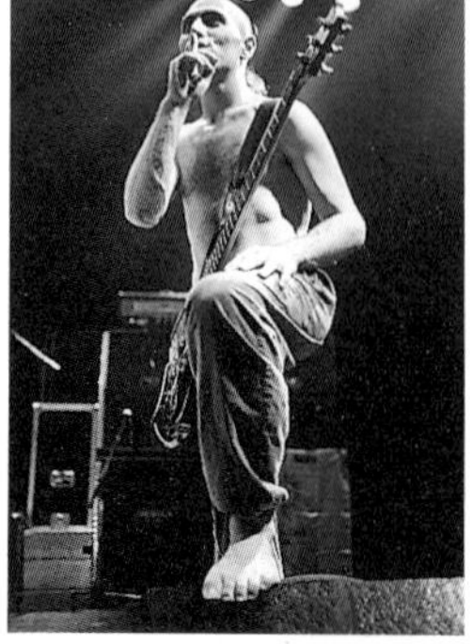

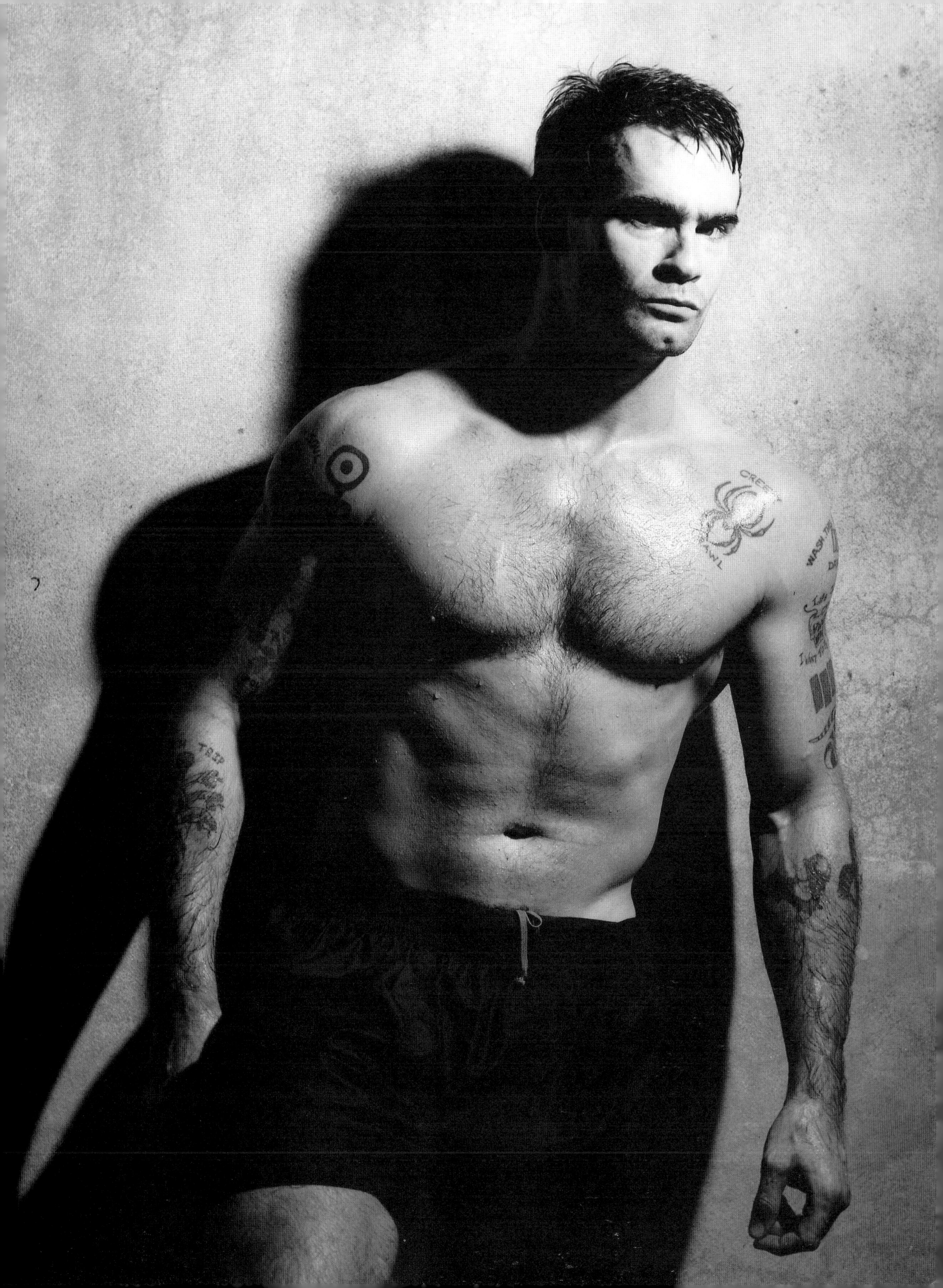

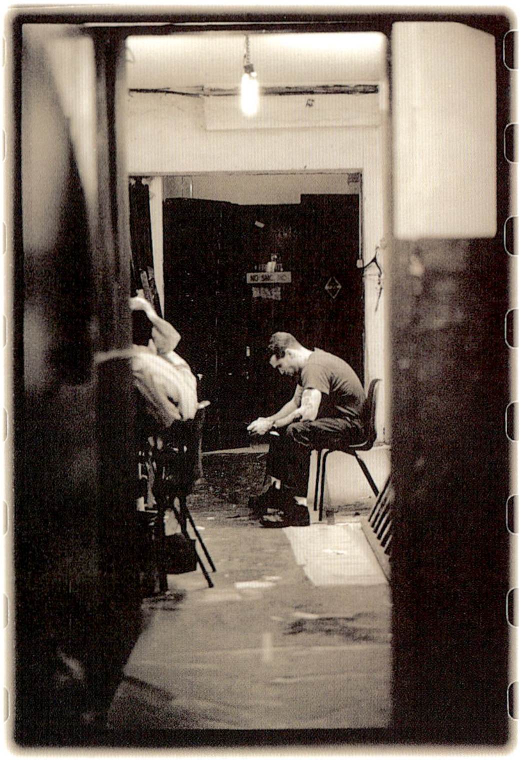

Henry Rollins
Dublin, '93

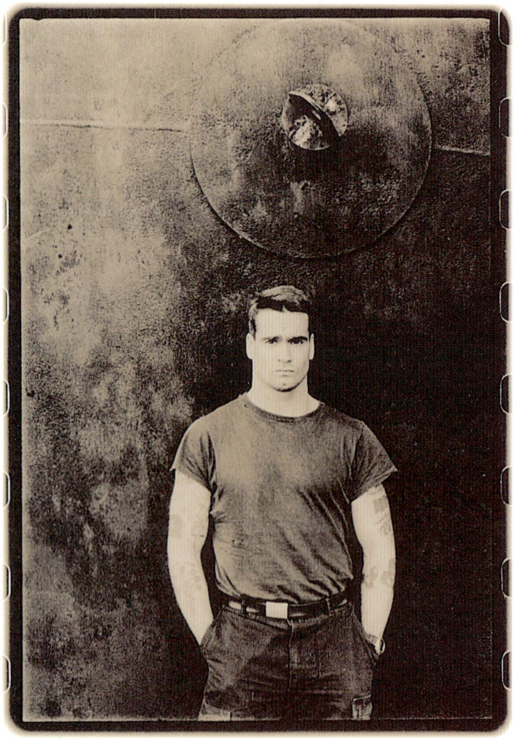

Right:
Greek Theater, San Francisco

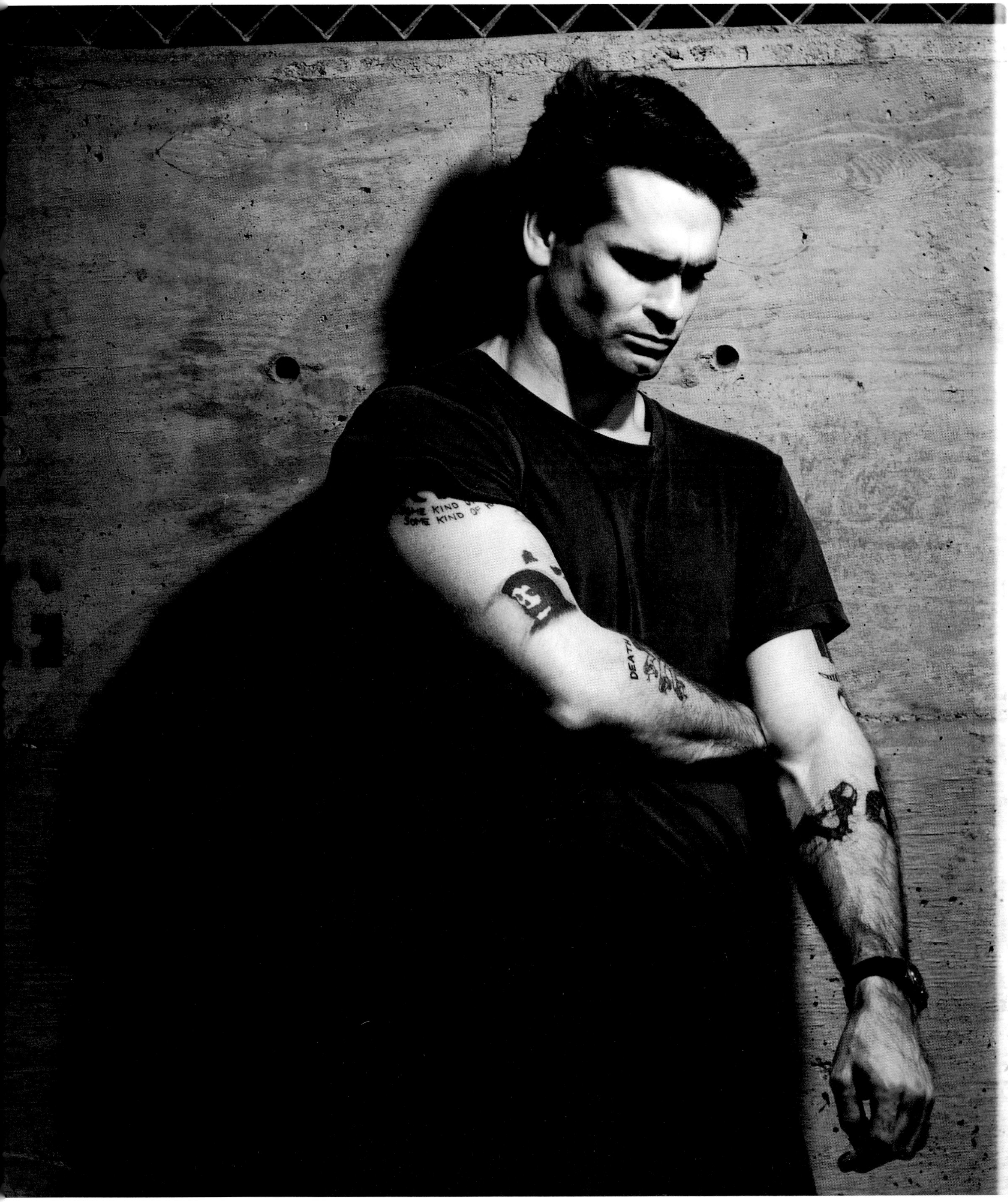
SOME KIND OF
DEATH

phil lynott
thin lizzy

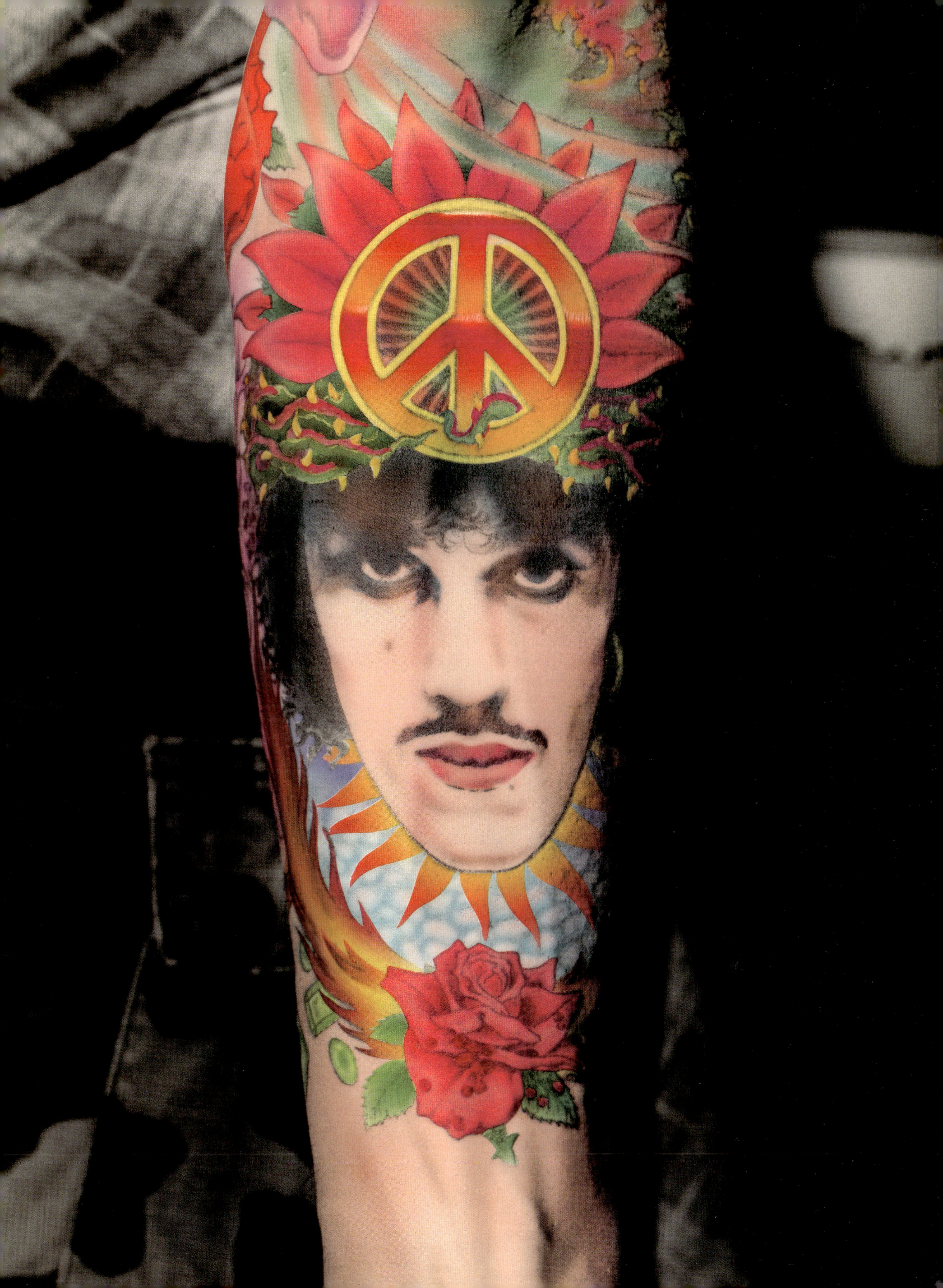

PHIL LYNOTT

THIS IS FOR ALL THE COWBOYS IN TOKYO

Phil is tired and his voice is forced. Phil is overweight and he's playing bum notes left and right. The keyboard player is covering. The rest of the band go through the motions laughing at each other as they make mistakes in every song. No one in the crowd seems to notice. Phil's face is broken and dull. Those close enough to know what's going on, know enough not to make comment lest they find themselves fired. It's such a long way from home. Phil says, "This is for all the cowboys in Tokyo." The crowd knows they're going to hear "The Cowboy Song". After that the band will probably slam right into "The Boys Are Back In Town" like they have so many nights before. "Are you out there Tokyo?" Phil hoarsely bellows at the crowd and you wonder if he can see them at all. Phil sounds so tired. They plod through the song and into "Boys". At the end of the song, the customary "the boys are back in town, get your knickers down" sounds violent, not the playful taunt of earlier tours. The beginning of the next number, "Suicide", starts with Phil telling the audience, "This is Brian's sayonara drum solo." A cold laugh follows and the band crookedly stumbles into the song. At the end of the song the set is over. The encore is rushed and uninspired. You can hear the misery in every note. At the end of the last song, Phil thanks everyone for coming and tells them that the band is going out for alcohol later. Phil is tired. The drummer's leaving. Another gig tomorrow night. Before that there's interviews to do, people to meet. Everyone wants to have their picture taken with him. He tries to be friendly but finds it hard. So far away from home.

HENRY ROLLINS

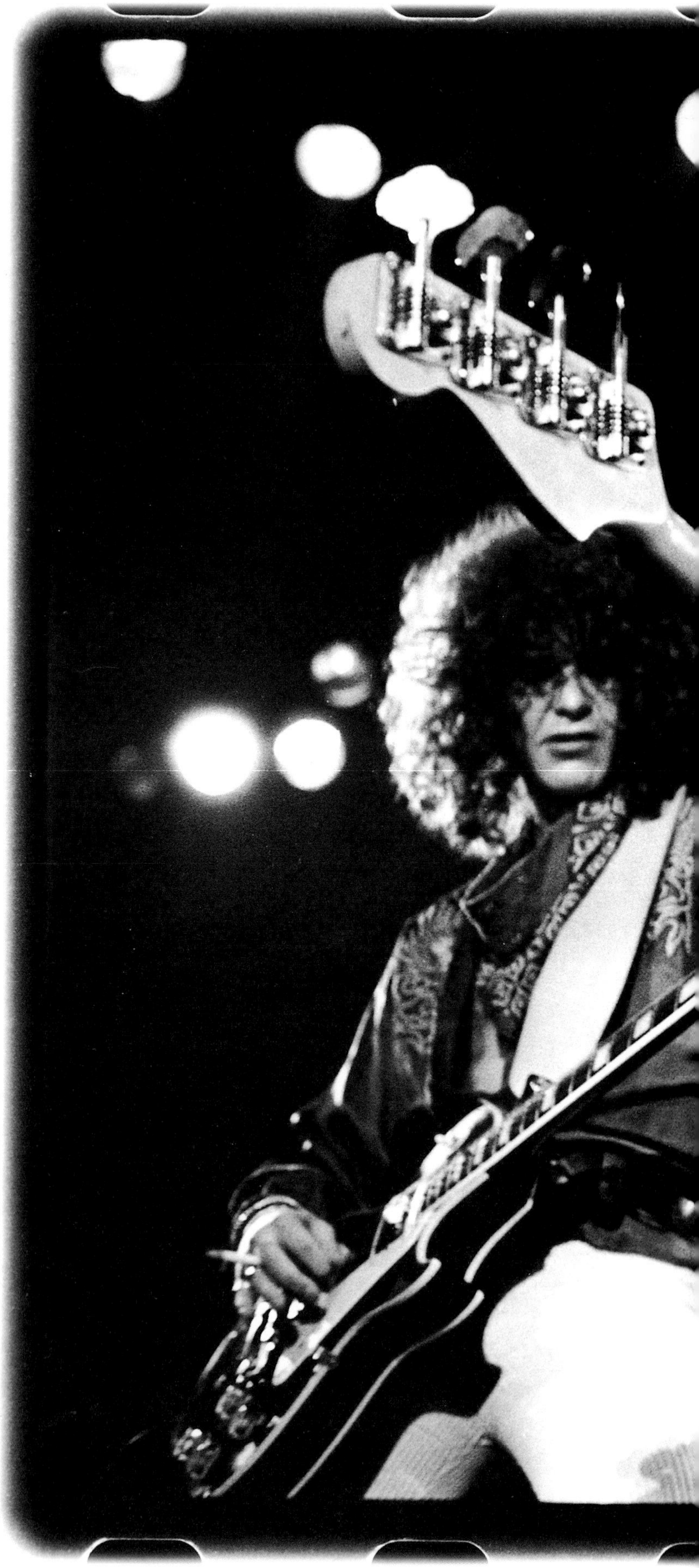

BRIAN ROBERTSON AND PHIL LYNOTT
BLACK ROSE TOUR
WEMBLEY ARENA

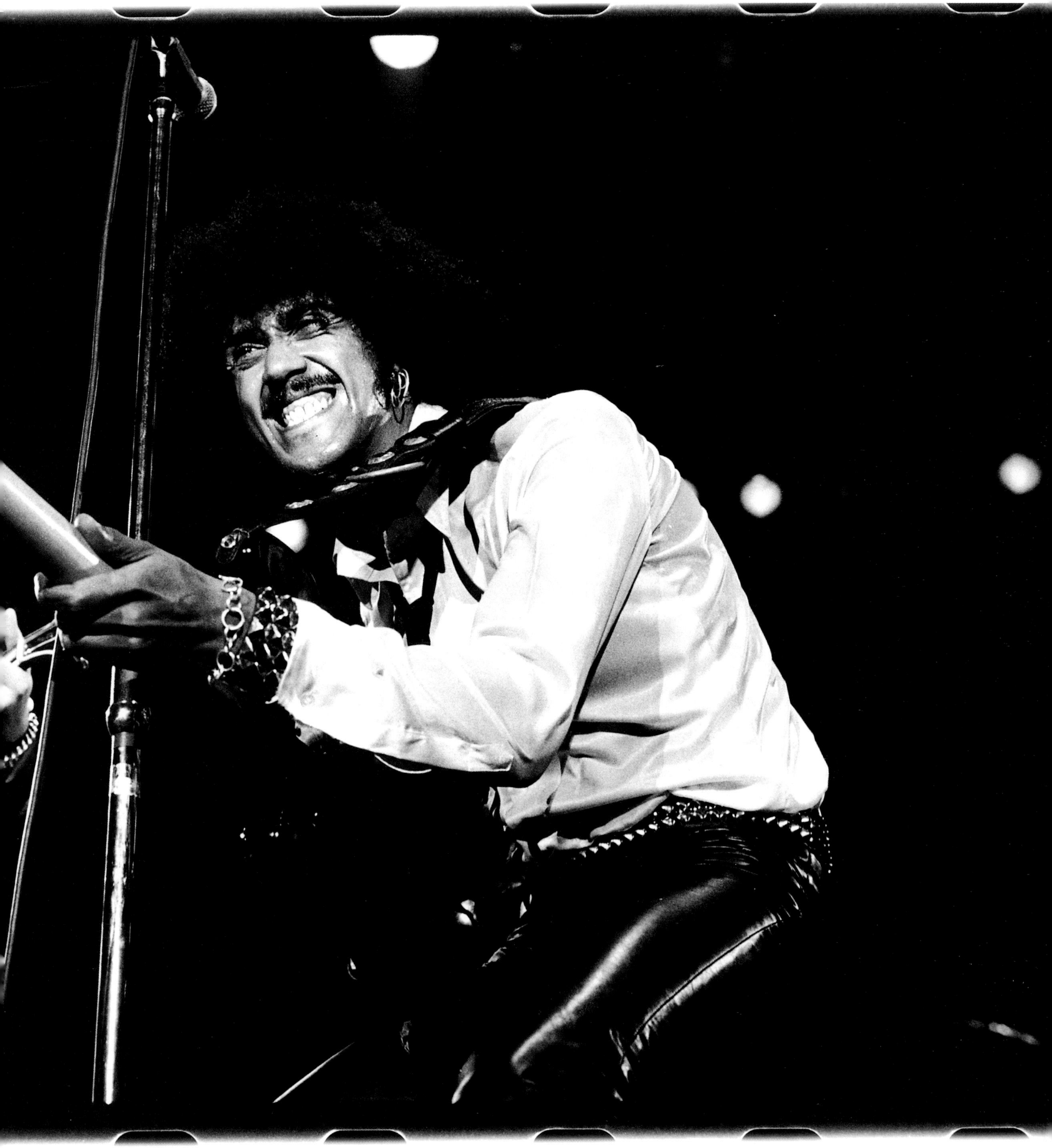

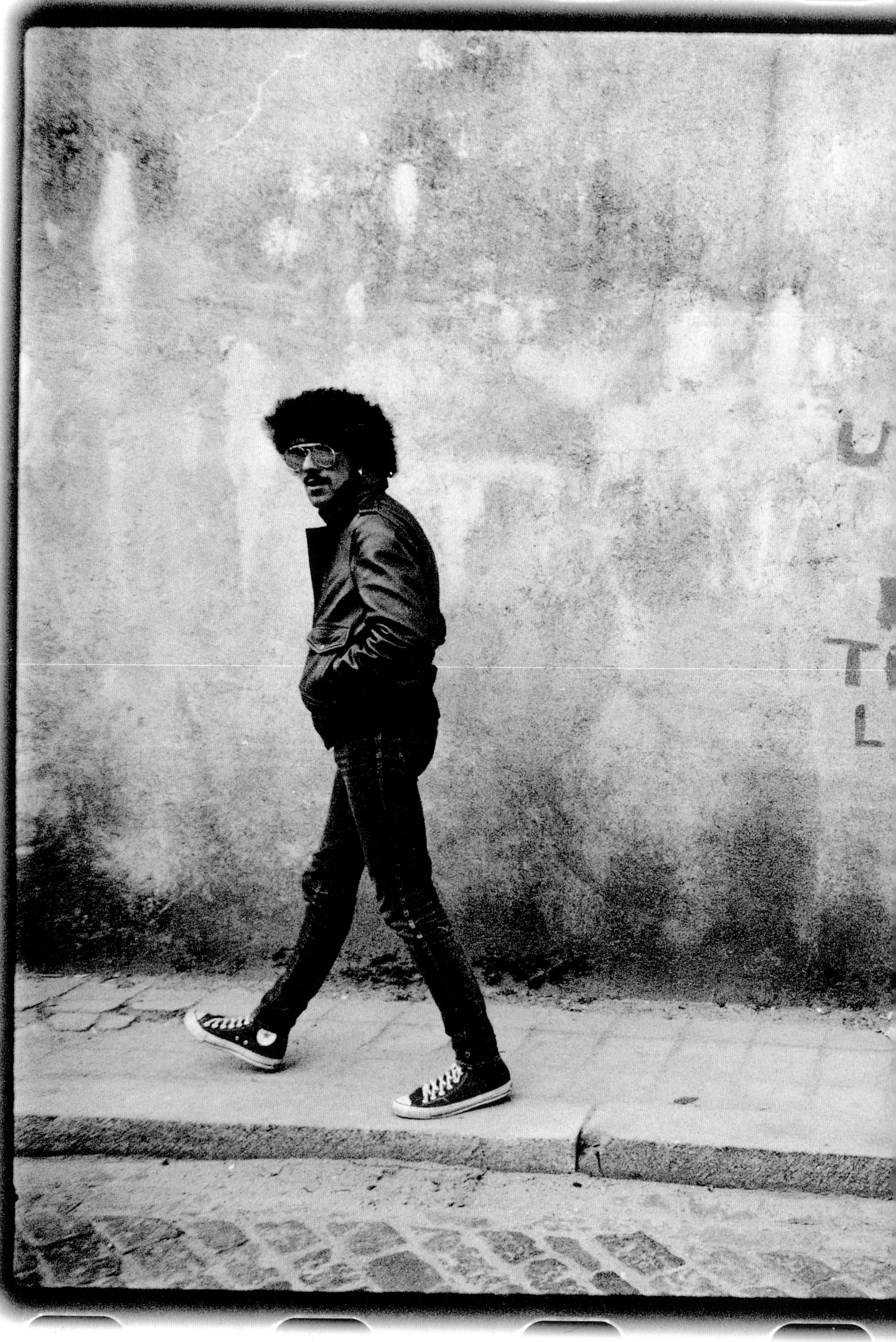

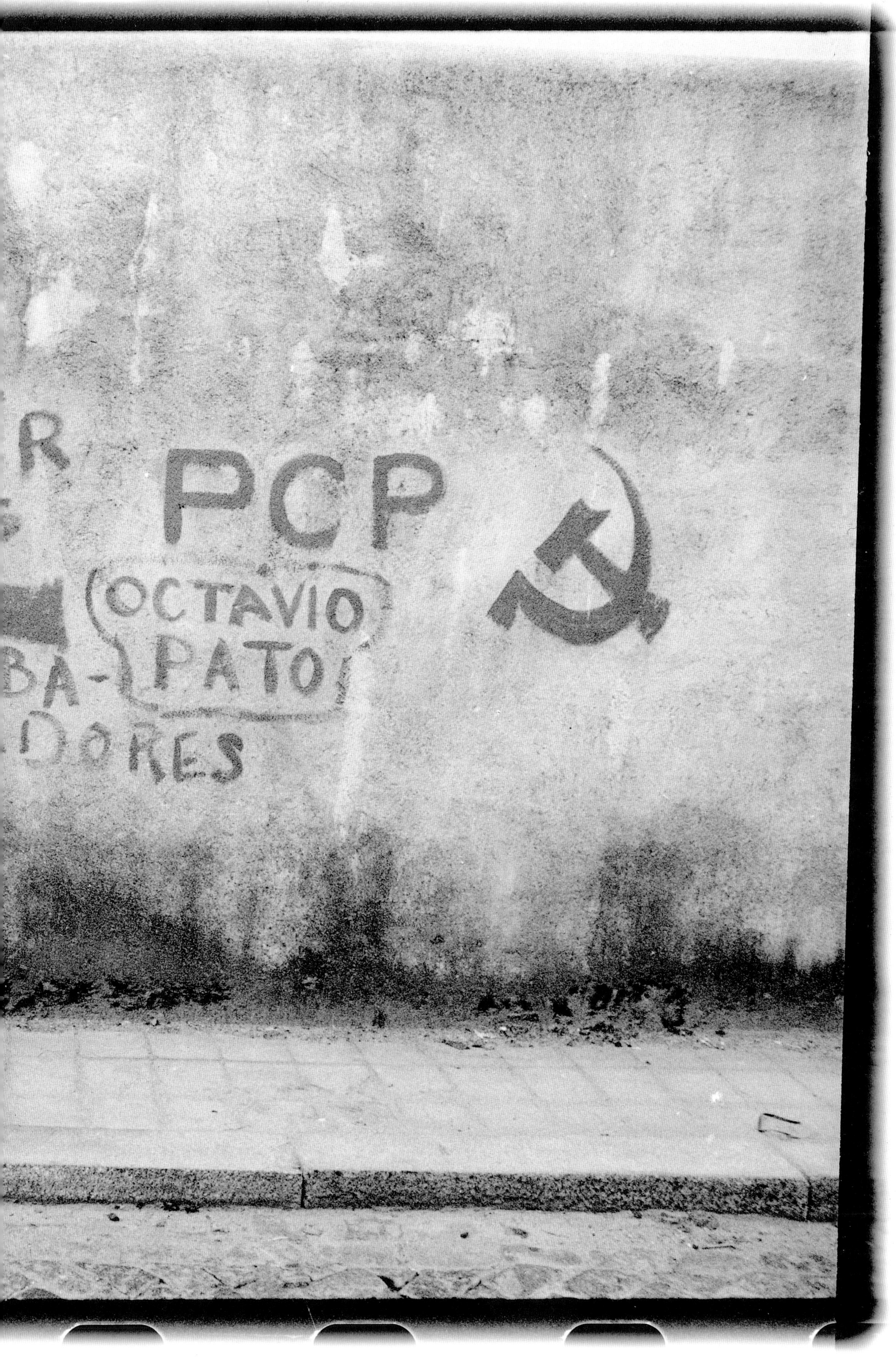
R
PCP
OCTAVIO
PATO
BA-
DORES

aerosmith

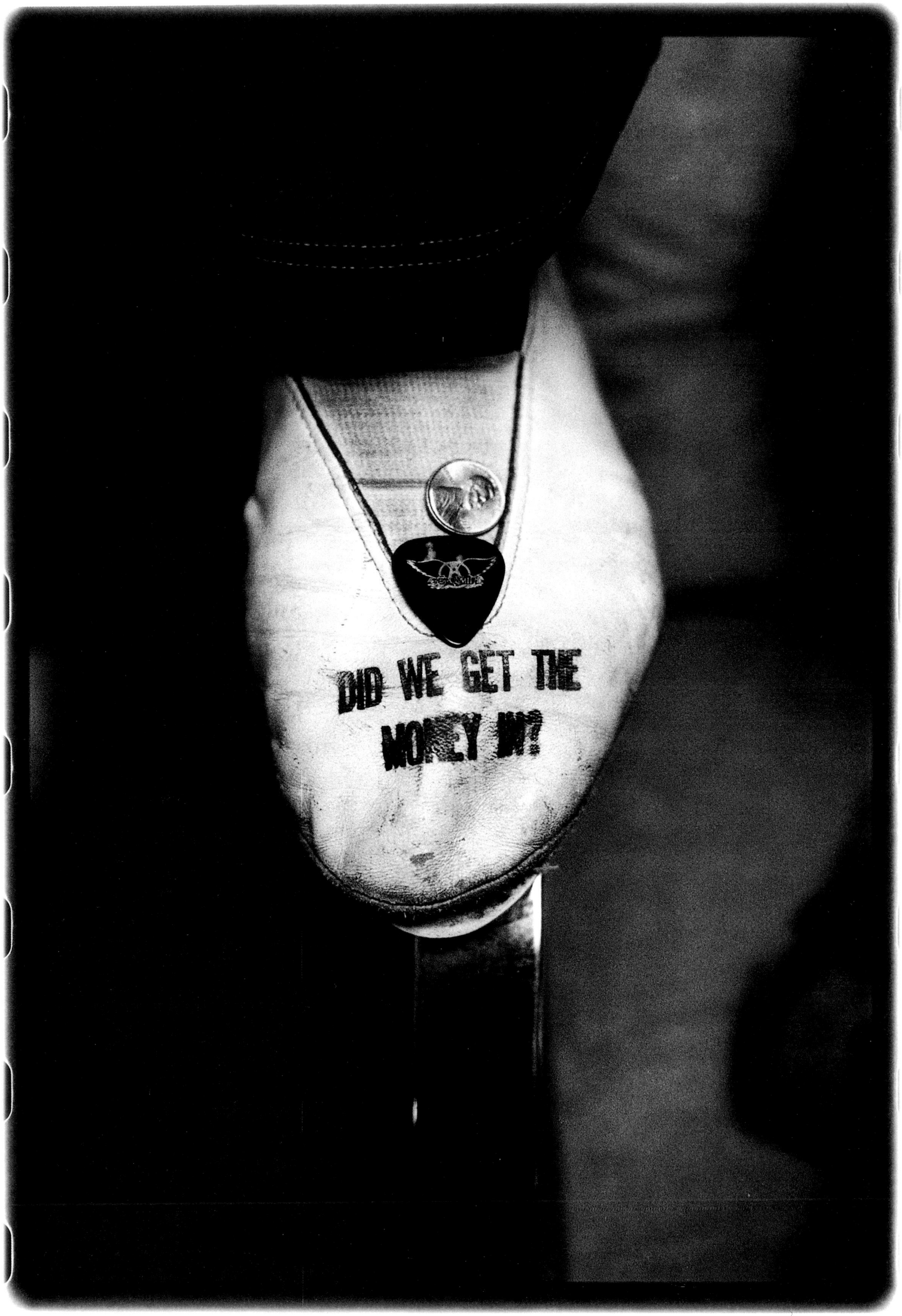
DID WE GET THE
MONEY IN?

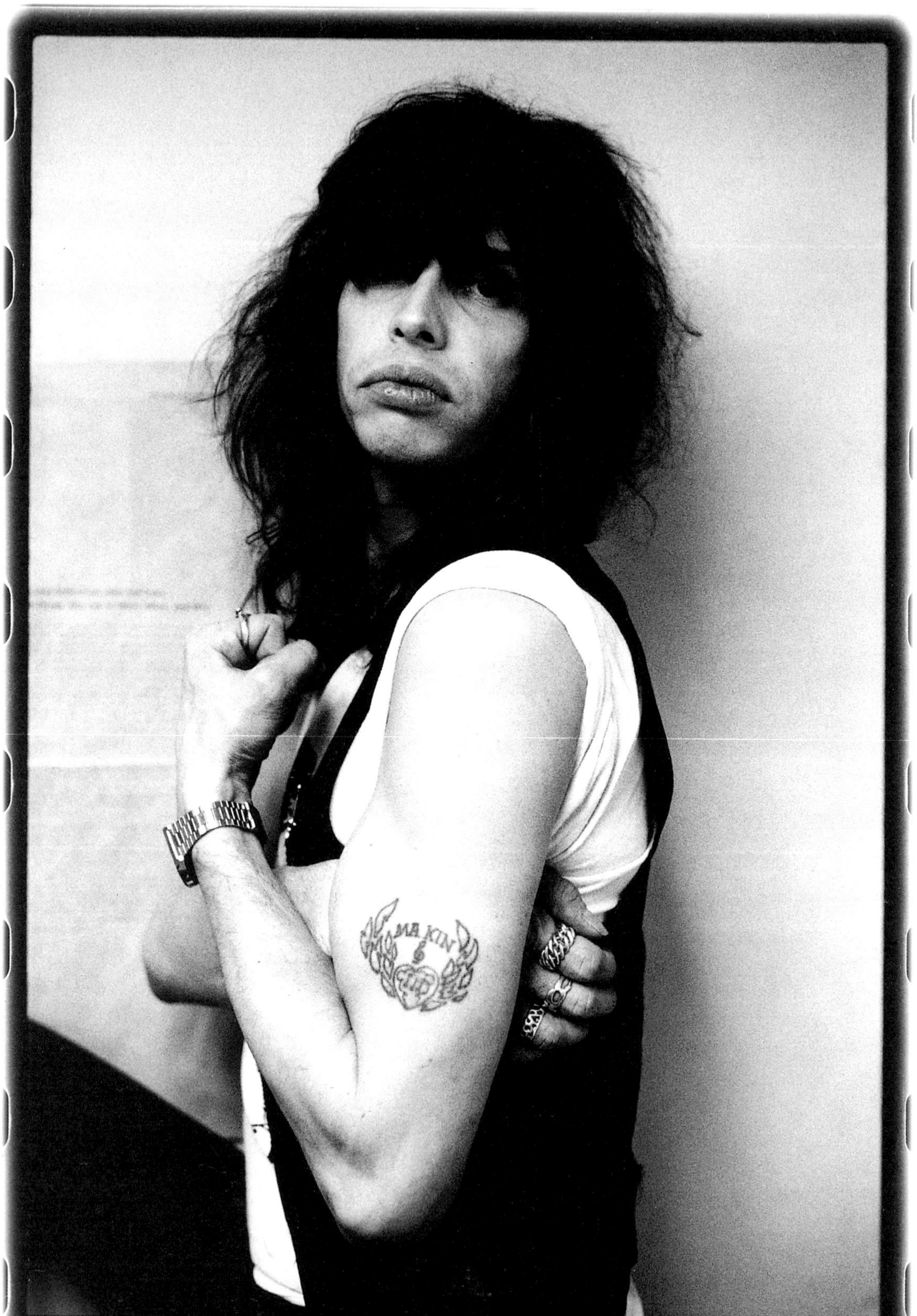

Steven Tyler
New York, '80

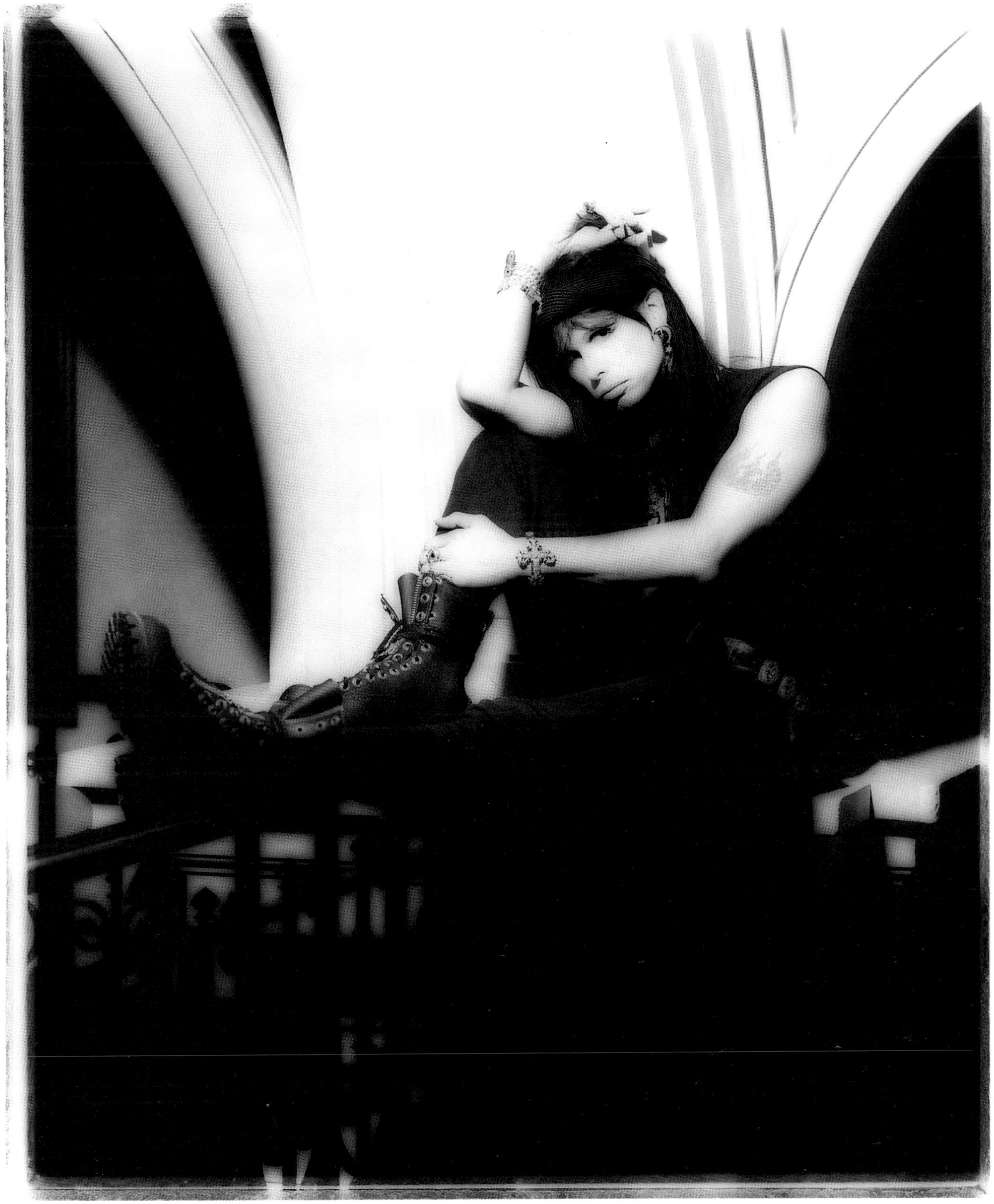

Steven Tyler
Paris, '93

AEROSMITH

THE WAY IT WUZ

In retrospect, the story is just a hazy blur of debauchery, excess and self abuse. But the actual facts remain crystal clear. It was around the time of Lennon's assasination, and New York was in the grips of the "Disco Sucks, Punk Rools" fiasco. At that time, Aerosmith were probably considered to be boring dinosaurs, along with all the other supergroups; old farts and has-beens that were vilified by the likes of Rotten and the rest of punks aristocracy (who in reality probably spent their teens wanking over Roger Dean covers and REO Speedwagon albums – you only need to look at Billy Idol to verify this fact). Anyways, my first encounter with the 'Smiths was in the early seventies; I reviewed their debut album and wrote them off as a bad imitation of the Stones who had got their image off a Queen album (then again, I also dismissed Kiss as an overnight sensation). Then I heard *Toys In The Attic* and got the message. Aerosmith were a band whose music I really dug but knew very little about. The more drugs I took the more I thought, "Hey wouldn't it be a gas hanging out with Tyler and Perry. Y'know, shooting the proverbial shit, listening to old R&B records, talkin' music and oh yeah! Taking loads and loads of high quality blow, surrounded by a posse of European looking babes avec high cheekbones and Biba style clothes. Fuck safety pins, self mutilation and cheap speed – this was high class fantasyland!

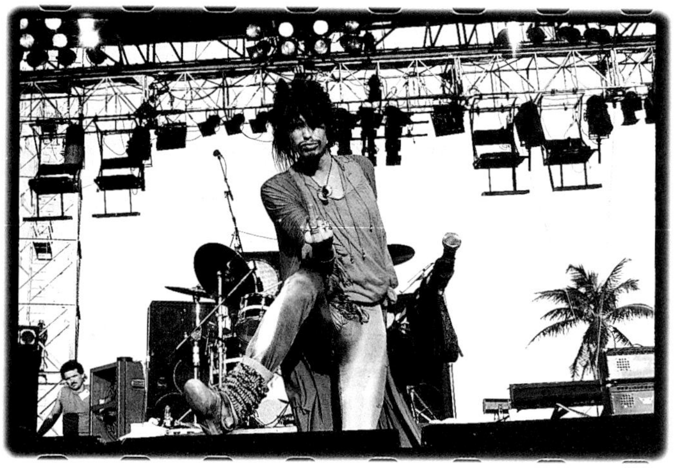

Anyways, it just so happened that Me'n'Ross were in New York under the pretense of covering some up'n'coming group, but in fact indulging ourselves in a binge of bourbon, drugs and extravagant room service bills courtesy of some desperate record company in search of the elusive front cover. Yes, I was a freeloader to the max, and abused my position of power. Nowadays when I reflect on my sorry past, I still look back on this period with fond affection. So there we were in the Big Apple, holed up in the flat of a drug buddy of ours, consuming vast amounts of coke, when the 'Smiths manager called us up and invited us over to the band's office, uptown. It was there I first set my eyes upon the reptilian visage of El Tyler. Looking stylishly gaunt with sunken pinned eyes, the man was a walking E chord, if you get my drift. He looked like he came out of the womb with silk Indian scarves wrapped around his umbilical chord. He was wasted and incoherent.

Frazzled, the man played us a selection of demos so loud that the speakers fell off the wall. We had to get an interview with him before he turned blue on us. Well, for obvious reasons, the management were a bit hesitant in letting us get an official audience with their prodigal stoned wastrel son. It was just by chance that one night at a comedy club, I came across his dealer – a female Jewish Princess NY style, a typical junkie friend/(fiend) of the stars, a fucking godsend, man. So after wining, dining, and bullshitting her into submission we arranged a secret rendezvous at the office in the wee early hours of the morning.

When we arrived, Tyler sat relaxed in a couch, with his new guitarist stooge at his side, lap dog fashion, and then ol' lady Serinda at his beck and call. If you've seen *Performance* then you would have really dug this scene. Tyler was a real gentleman and in his opiated stupor entertained us with his old videos of the band (the one that stands out featured Little Richard on 'Bandstand') and anecdotes (like the time Tyler took some amyl nitrate on a big dipper with Jimi Hendrix, I mean how fuckin' cool can you get?) I knew very little about the band factually, but it didn't matter as we were all shitfaced and I never got to write the story anyway. We finished off the evening with Ross taking a picture of The Man holding up a giant Quaalude cushion made by a fan. A fitting end to a 24 carat rock'n'roll evening. Now many moons have passed, Tyler is clean and sober and the original Aerosmith are back together. I still couldn't name you a toon off their last four albums.

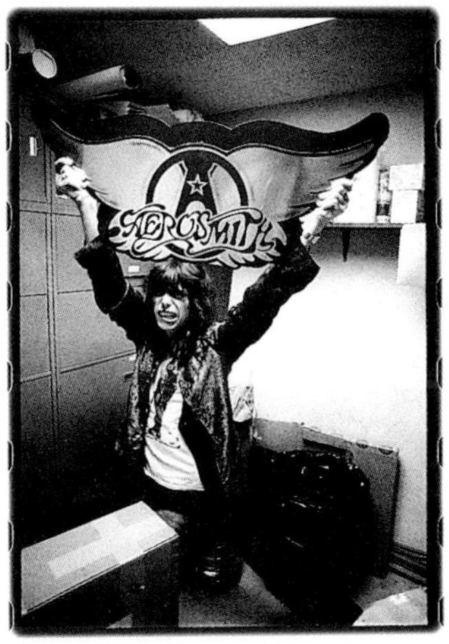

Don'cha just love happy endings?

PETE MAKOWSKI

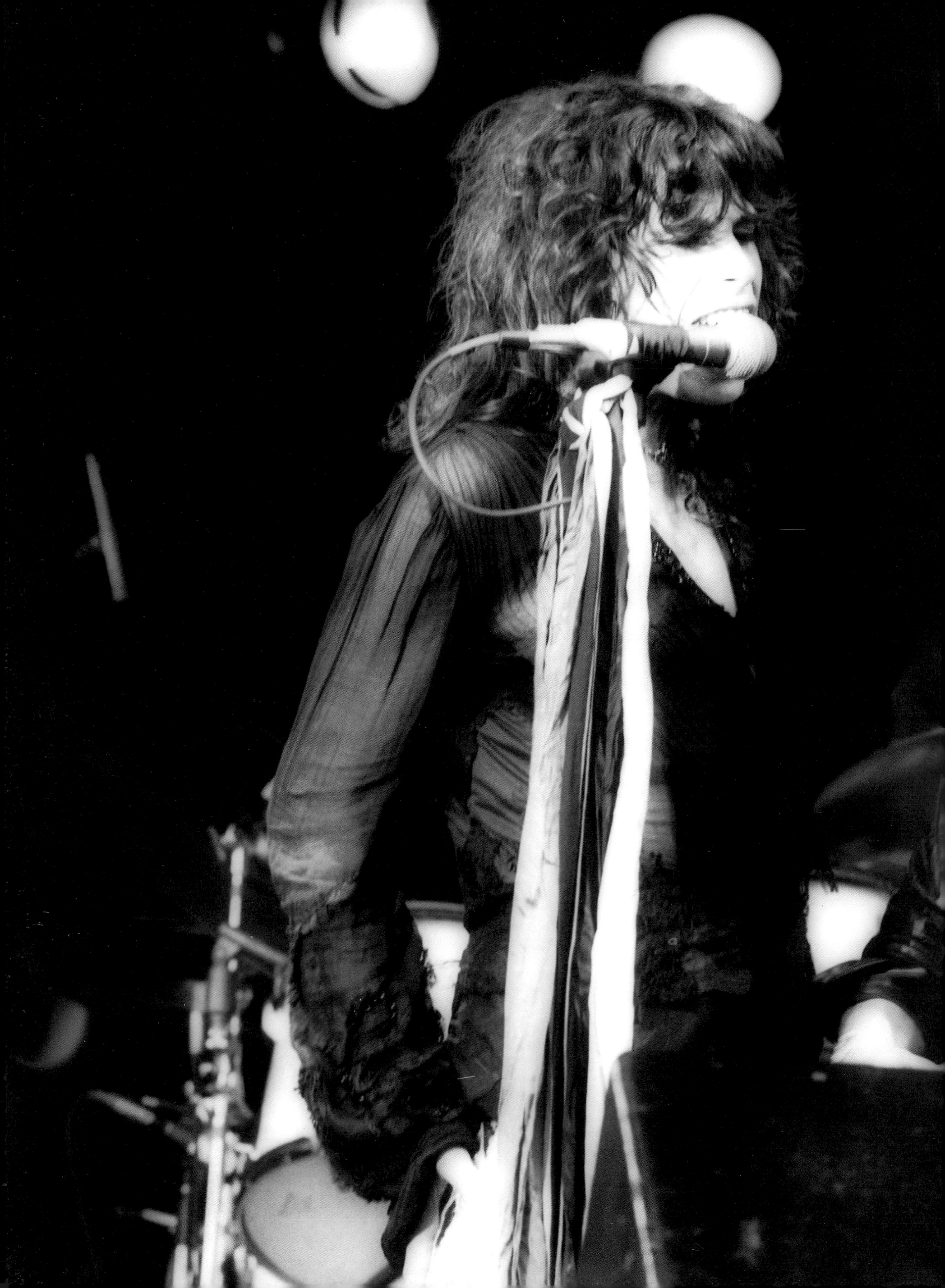

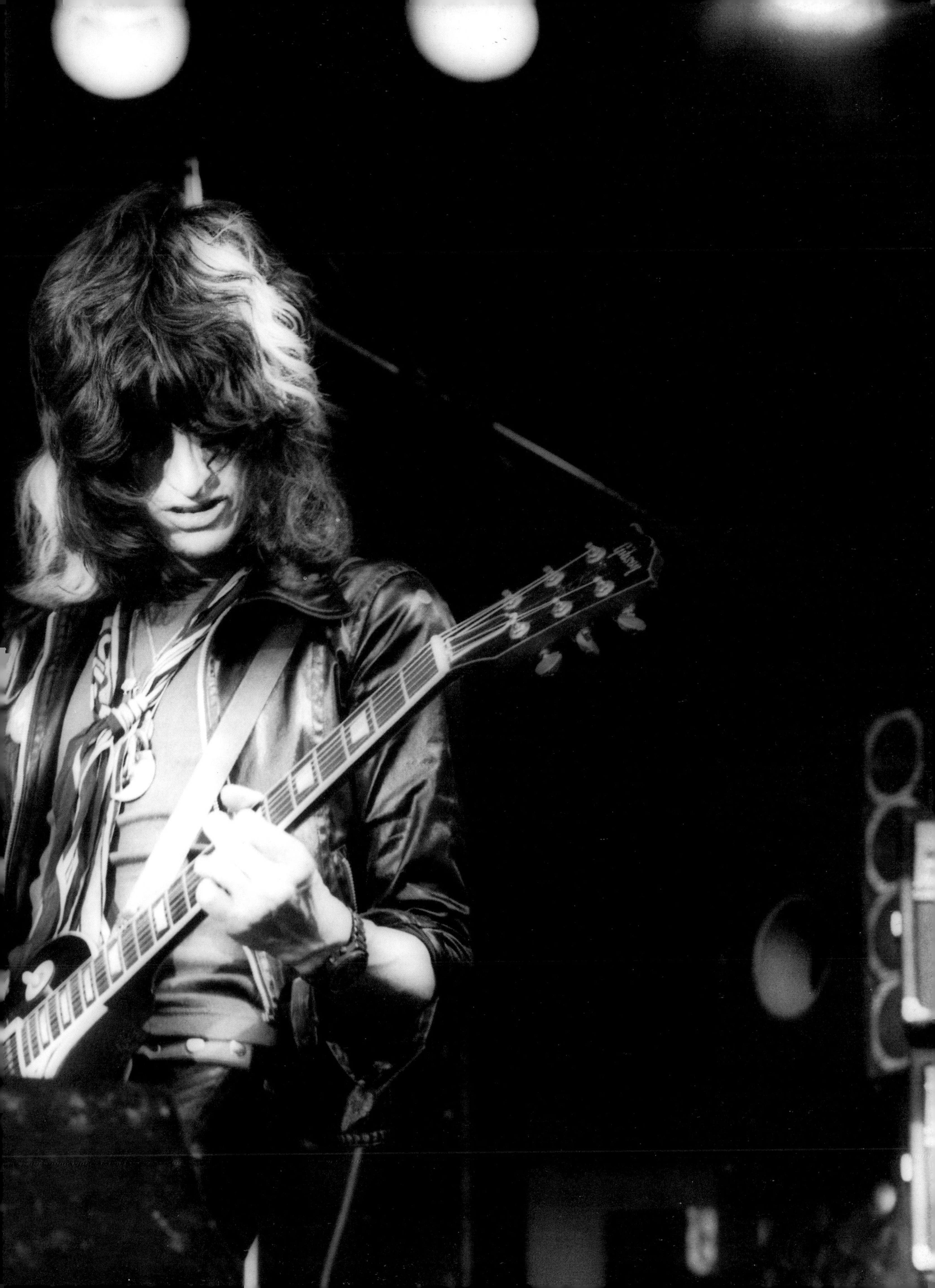

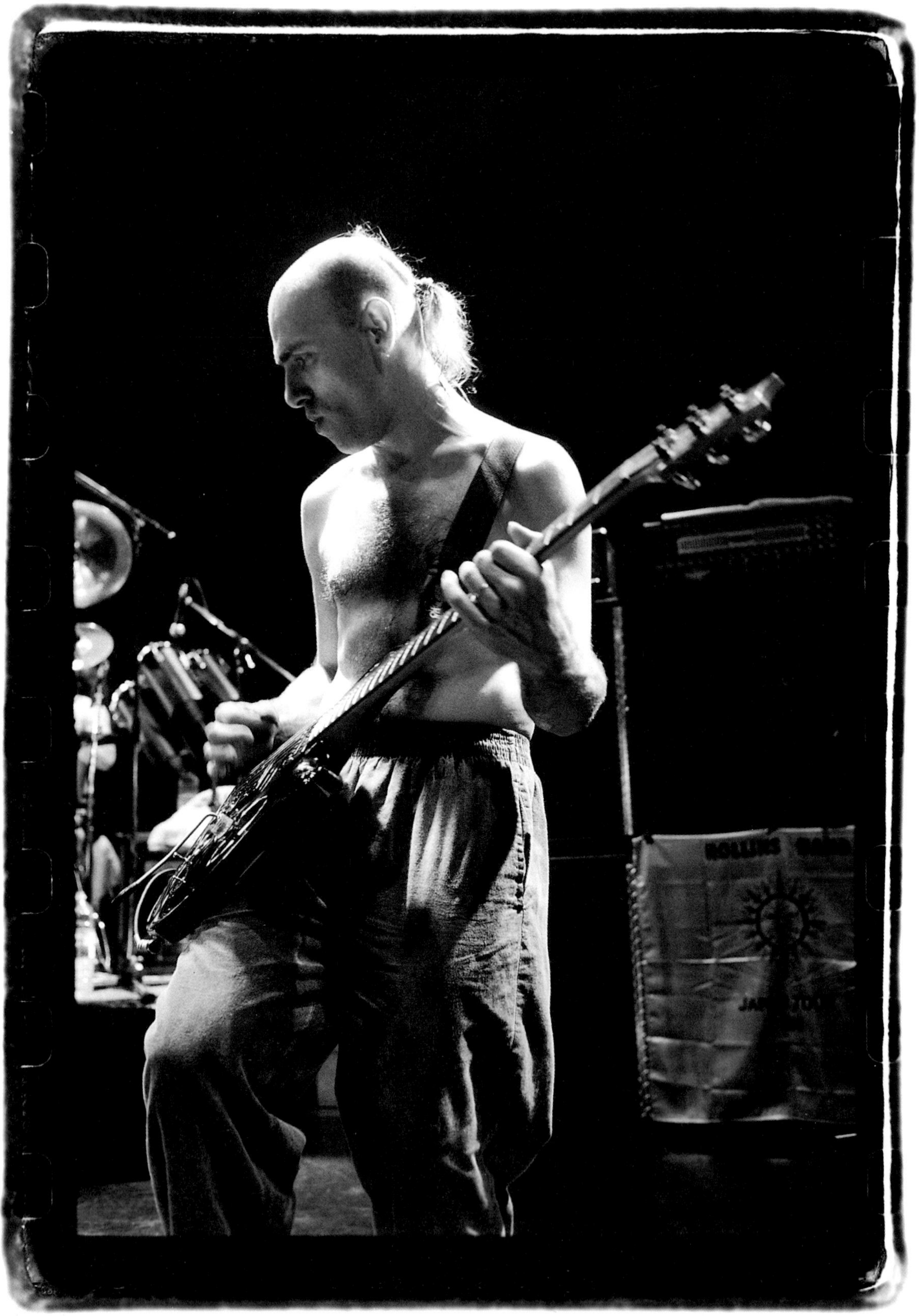

Chris Haskett
Tokyo, '94

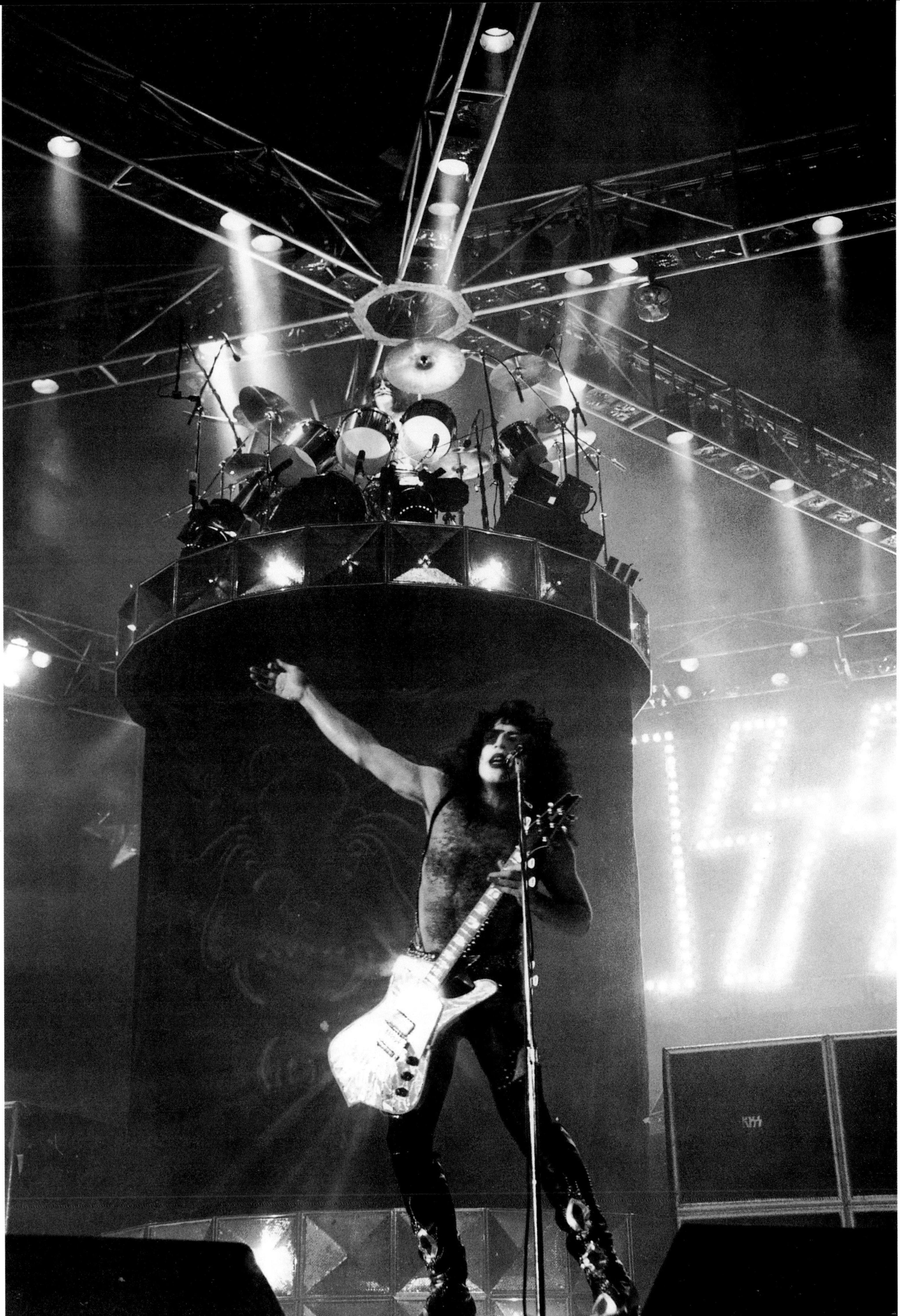

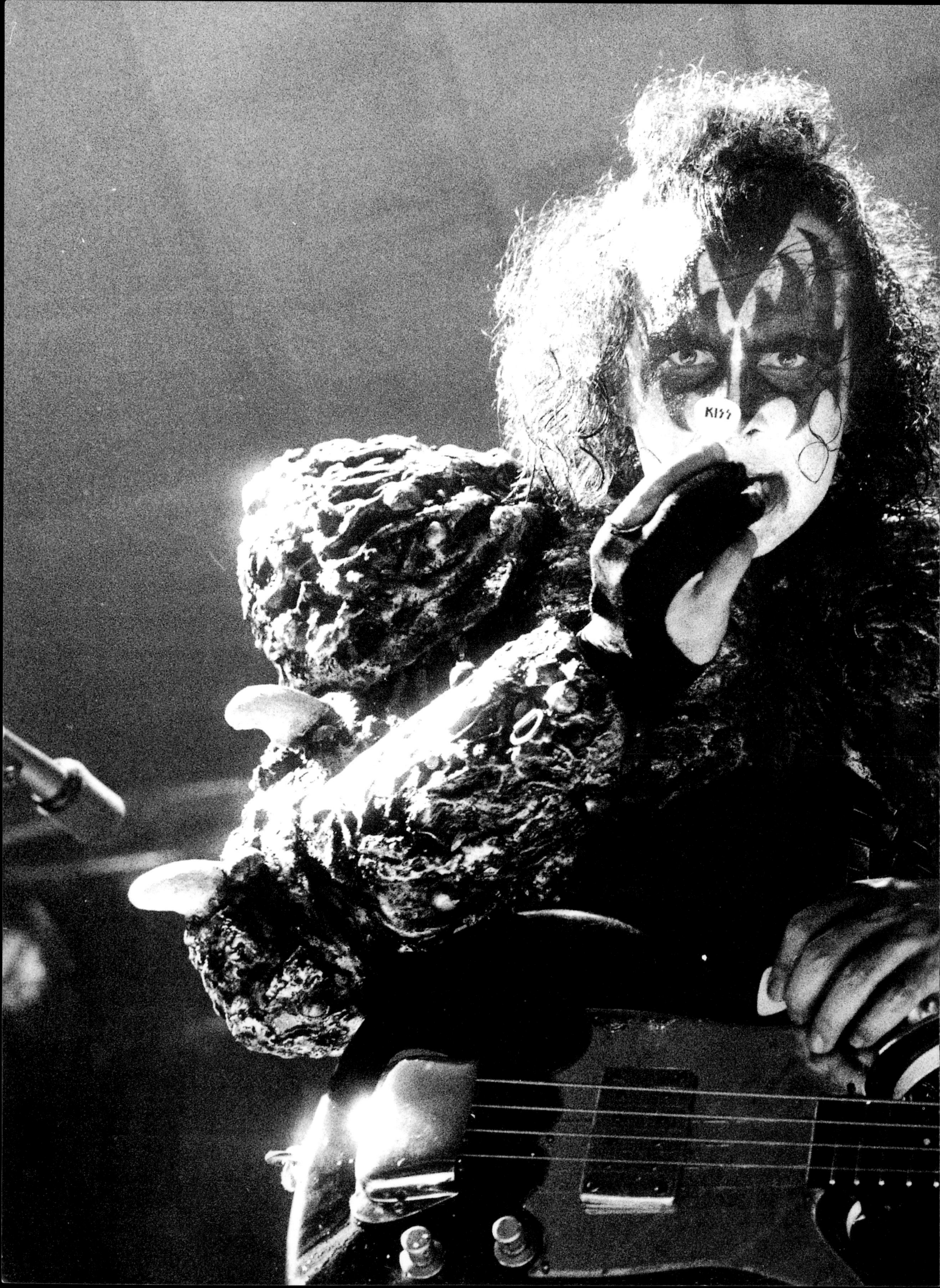
KISS

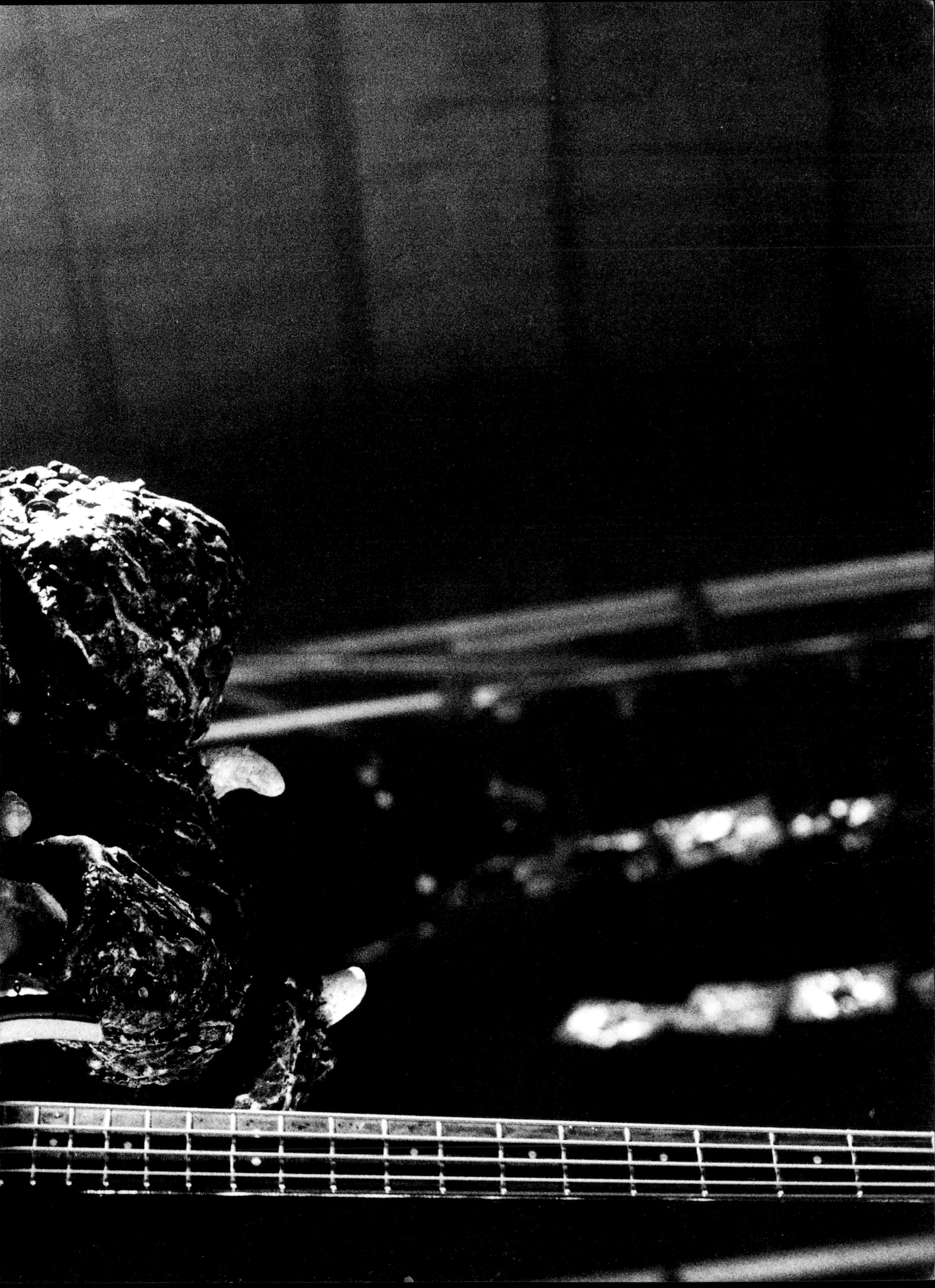

pete townshend

Pete Townshend
Concerts For Kampuchea
December 28, 1979

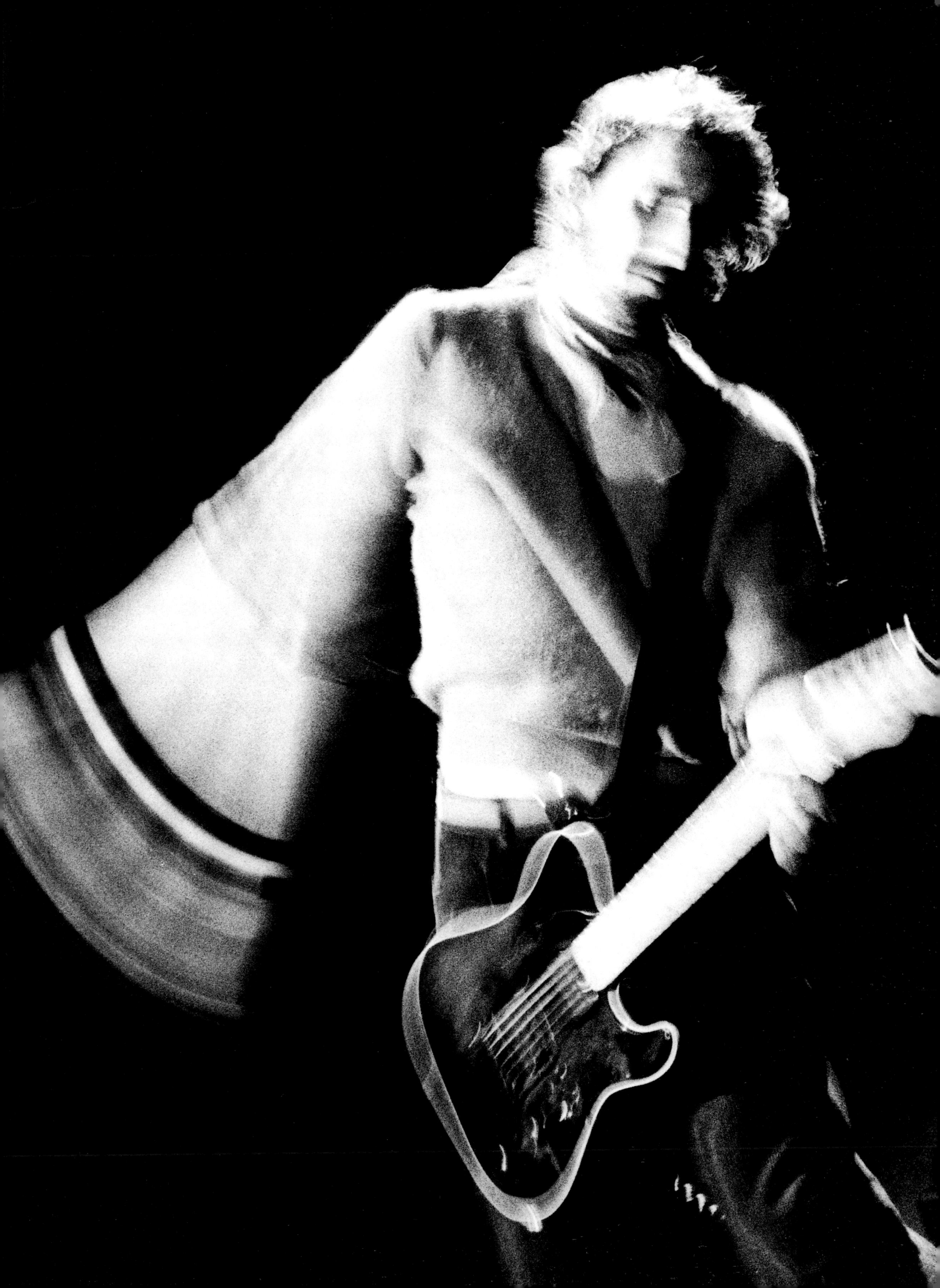

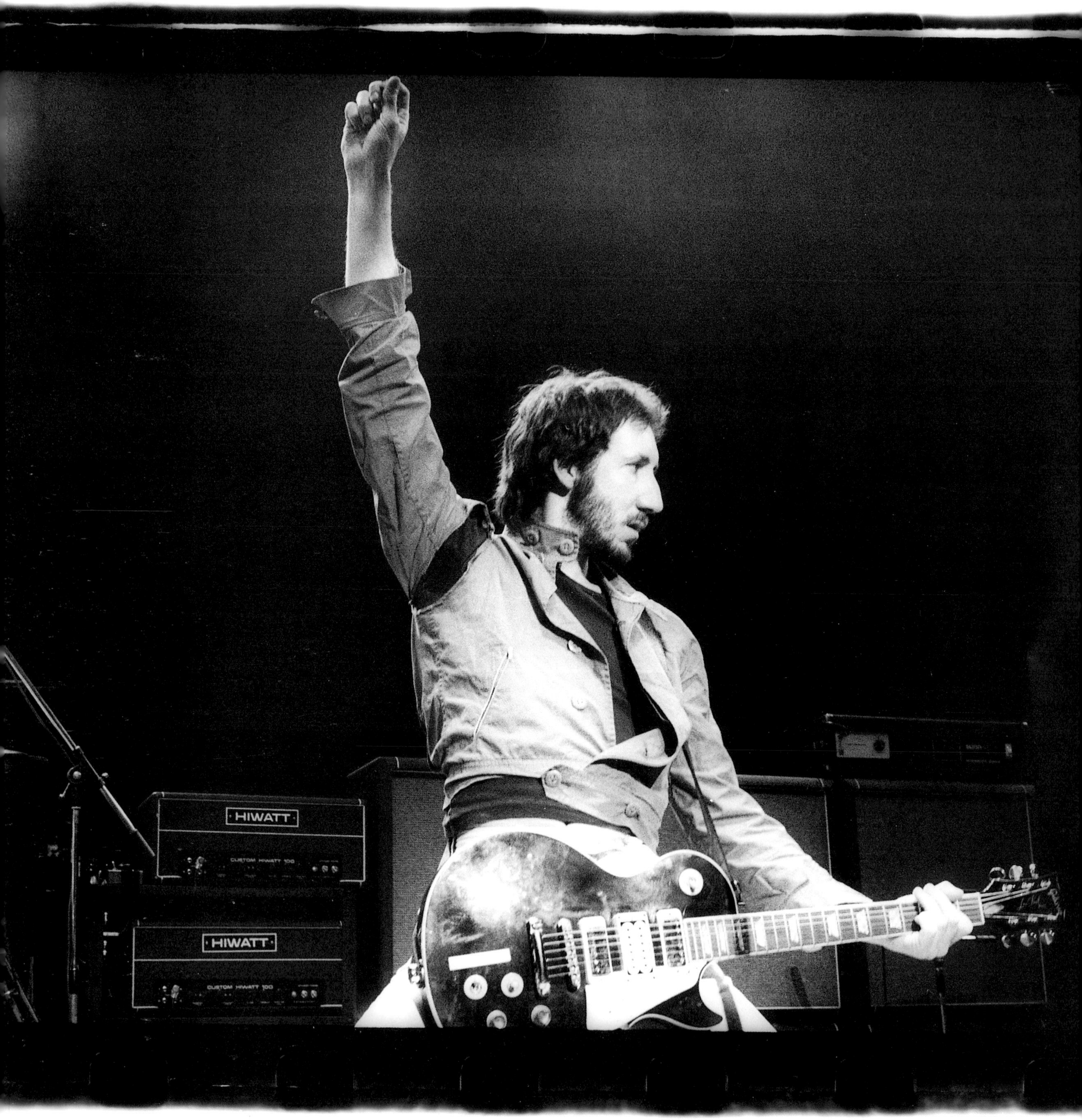

Pete Townshend, Shepperton, May 25, 1978

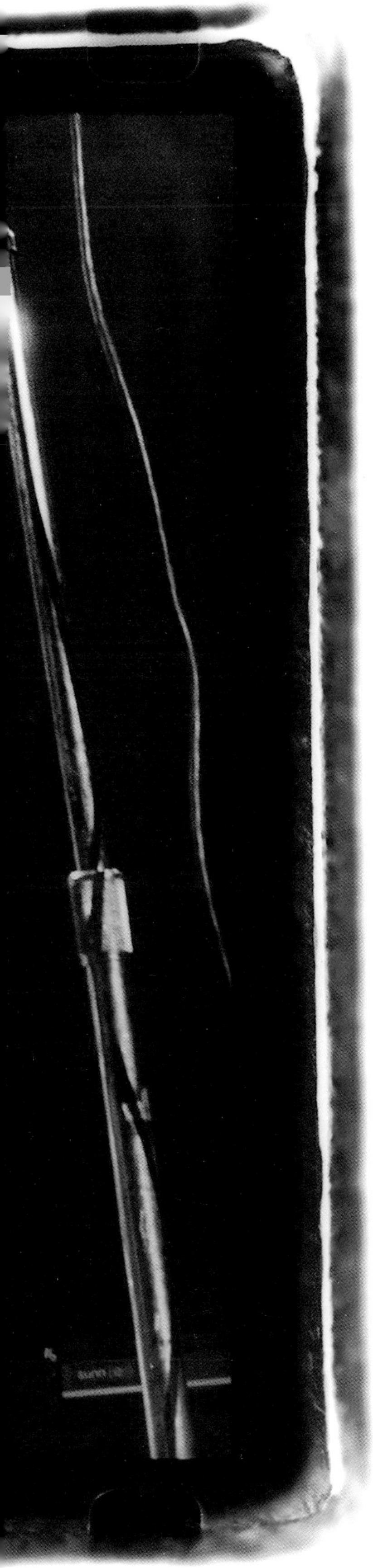

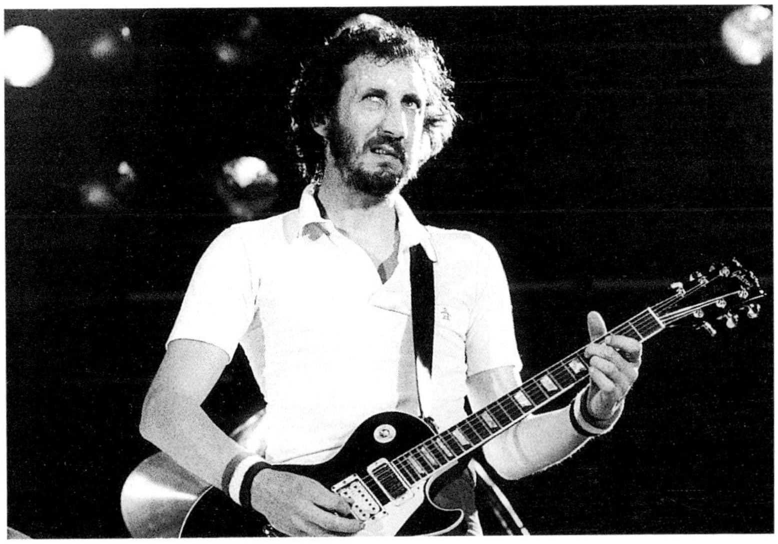

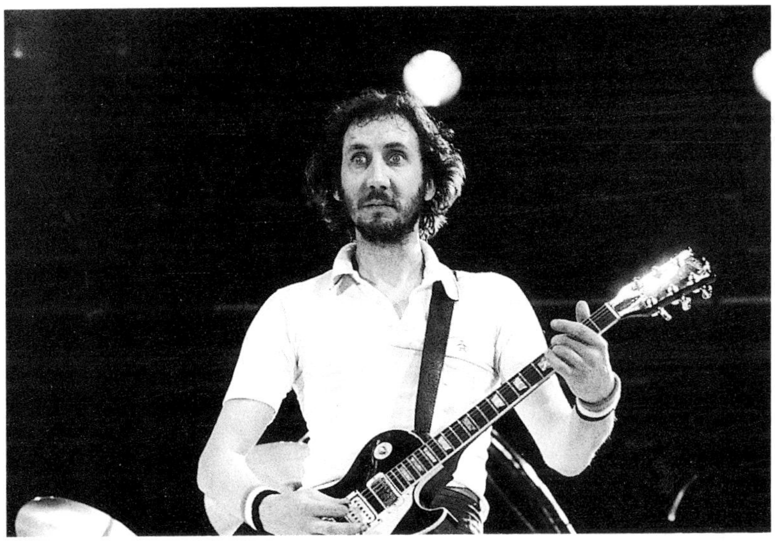

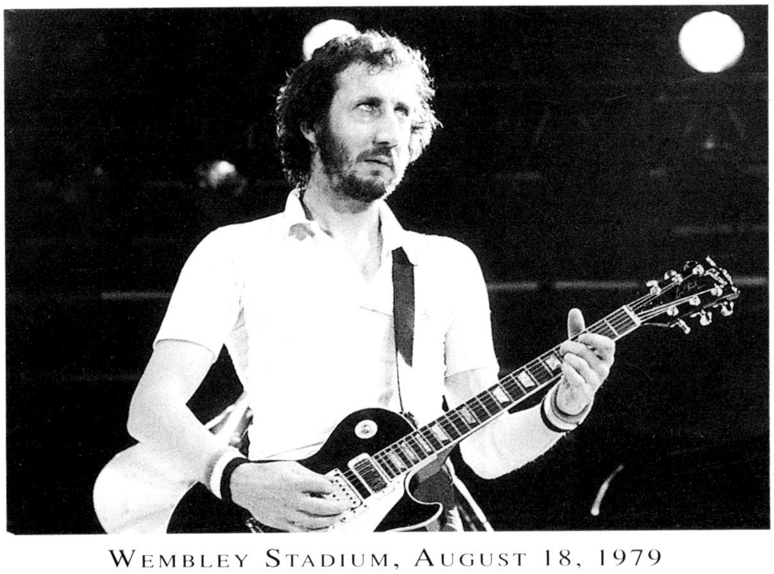

Wembley Stadium, August 18, 1979

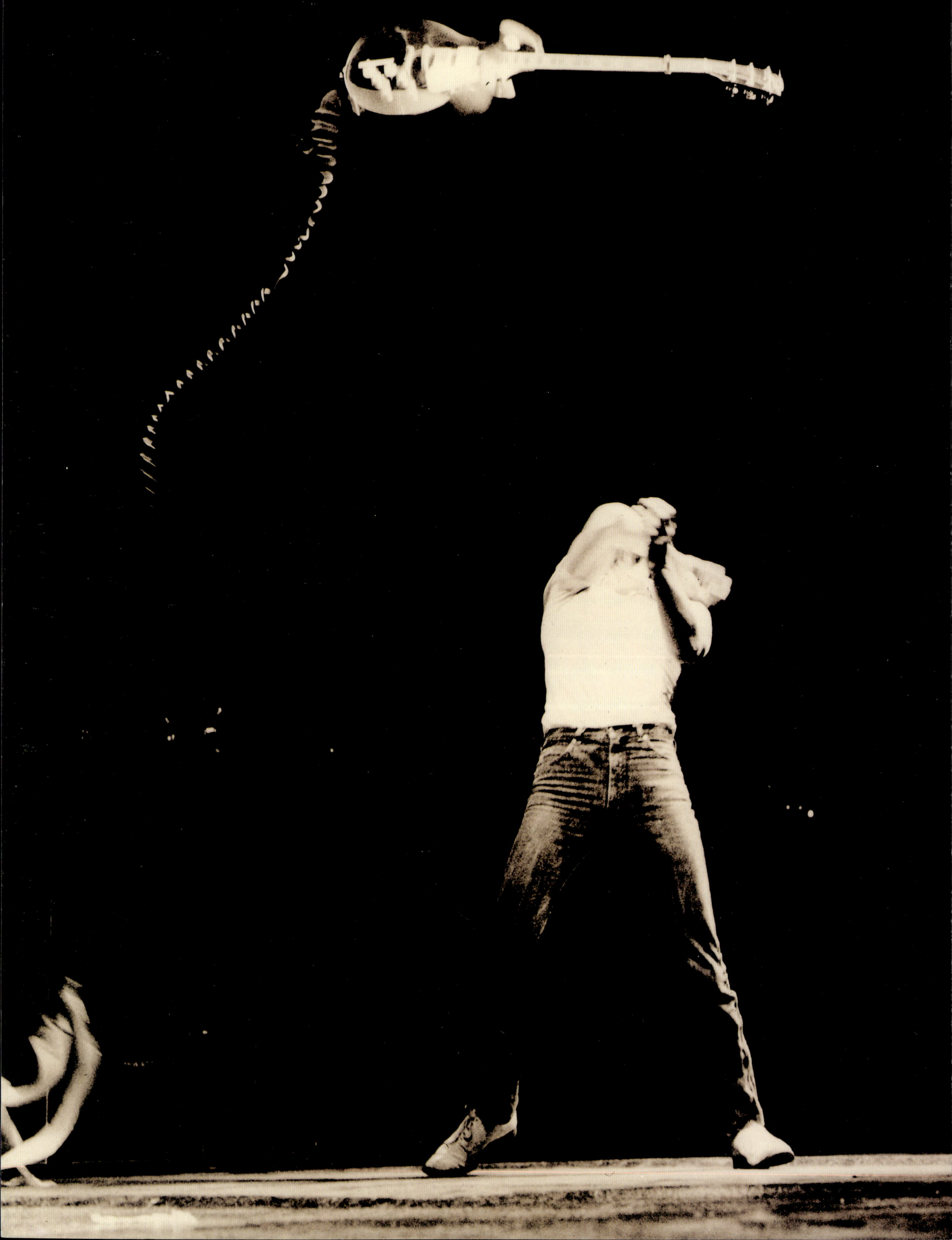

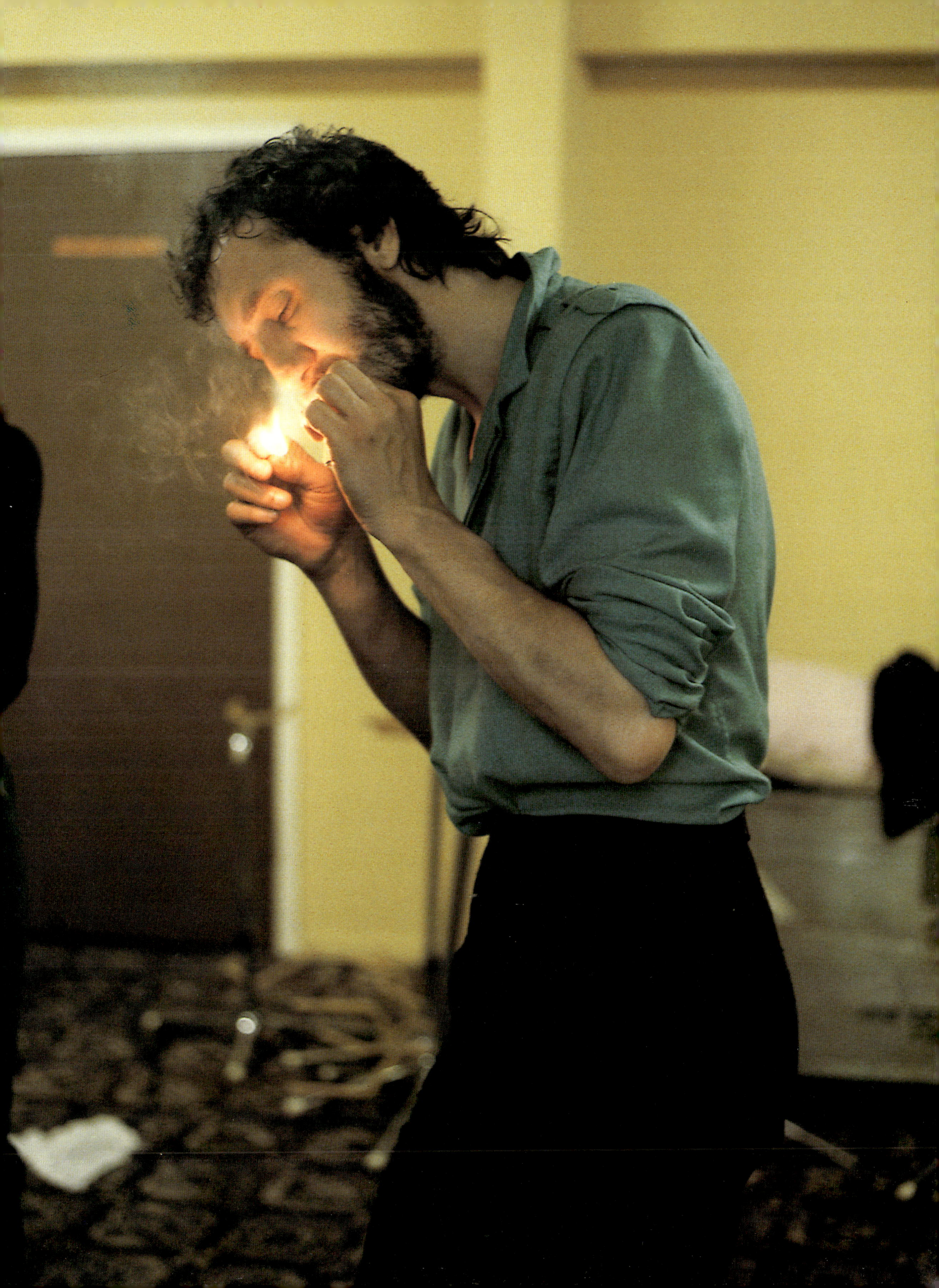

PETE TOWNSHEND

I originally wanted Linda Walker (a big Who fan) to write something on them for my book. She hummed and ah'd and then said, "I don't like them anymore." "So write about that," I said. Her reply: "I couldn't bring myself to. I couldn't let them down like that."

She's still a fan.

I didn't discover The Who until '70 when I got *Live At Leeds*. I didn't discover *Tommy* until a mate at Scouts told me to get it. The first time I ever saw them live was at The Oval, September 18th, 1971 - I was 14. It was the British premiere of The Who's next tour.

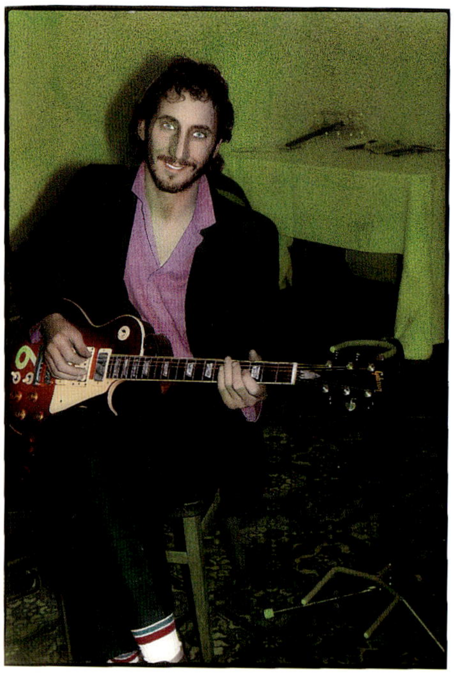

On the '73 tour, I queued for 11 hours to get tickets to see them at The Lyceum. I was trying to impress my girlfriend Michelle Green. On the night of the show, I took her down to the front of the dance floor and when they came on, we got completely crushed. After the third number, we had to leave because she was hysterical and in tears. To this day, I've never really forgiven her. To make up for it, when The Who played at the Sundown Edmonton in December, I got tickets and took her to the final night, December 23, '73! I remember halfway through "Magic Bus" being told to please stop standing on my seat because I was embarassing her.

I saw them a lot in the 70s – both Charlton shows, Wembley '75, Hammersmith Christmas shows '76 - I still have all the tickets. I mention this because I want you to understand how much The Who meant to me as a teenager.

The reason I became a photographer in the first place was that after seeing The Who at Wembley in '76, I decided to forget about the BA degree in Art I was studying for and to start taking pictures of The Who.

I first officially shot them on May 25, '78 at Shepperton Studios during the filming of *The Kids Are Alright*, (the last show ever with Keith Moon). I got to meet Keith at a party I was photographing for the Steve Gibbons Band. I had dropped 6 tabs of speed and cornered him for an hour. I must have bored the arse off him, but he was most charming and gracious and I remember coming away thinking "What a great bloke."

Looking back, the main thing I remember about the early 80's is that I went right off The Who. I still had the fondness that all true fans have for their first love, so to speak, but thought that Townshend had become a sad hero to worship. It was a shame, I didn't even like his solo albums much. It wasn't his fault though - we were both getting older.

Then after several years of not giving a shit, a friend of mine got me front row seats for the show at the Albert Hall in October '89. I spent the first half of the show within jumping distance from Townshend and Daltrey and was so in awe, I had to go to the bar at the intermission to have a few drinks. It was a nice surprise to discover how I could still relate to a band I cared about as a teenager and The Who are still the greatest fucking rock band I've ever seen - and, believe me, I've seen most of them.

Inevitably, I suppose, I finally got round to taking some solo shots of Townshend. It was in Los Angeles, during his solo tour in August '93. I was shooting the Wiltern Theater shows for Bill Curbishley (The Who's manager). I

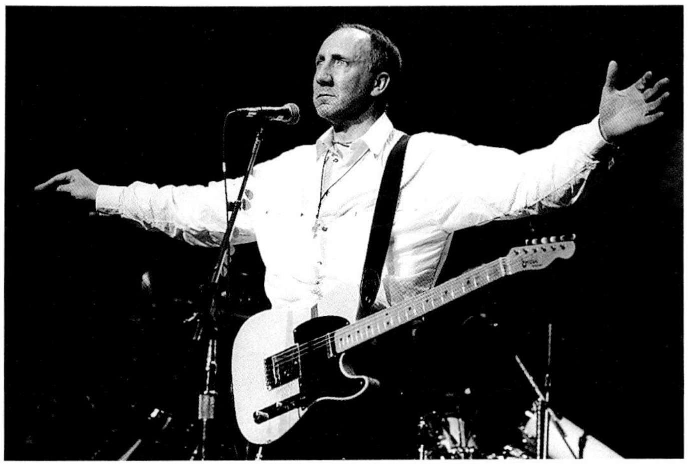

Pete Townshend, '93

shot the first show and afterwards, Bill said, "Why don't you come back and say hello to Pete? I've been telling him about you." So I went up to Townshend, who looked really knackered, leaning up against his dressing room wall and said, "Hi, I'm Ross," and he looked at me really blankly - it was obvious that Bill hadn't said a word to him - he was just trying to help out. Anyway, to make up for it, Bill arranged for me to do some solo shots of Townshend. He was doing the Jay Leno show at Universal Studios where I was told to meet him. I got there early, of course, and Townshend turned up about 2 hours late, looking thoroughly miserable. I went to approach him and he blanked me and went into his dressing room. Eventually, Nigel (his minder) told me to go in and just ask him straight, "Do you want to do any pictures today or not?" So I did. Townshend was pacing up and down, saw me come in, and yelled, "Get out of my fucking dressing room, go on, now and stop fucking lurking, just go away!" As I left, Nigel said, "Oh, sorry mate." I said, "Look, why don't you find out if he wants to do this and I'll wait downstairs." Fifteen minutes later – there he was, my hero. I was pleased, but nervous. There he was, completely stone faced, chewing gum and looking as miserable as only he can manage. I started taking pictures and got 20 minutes out of him in the end.

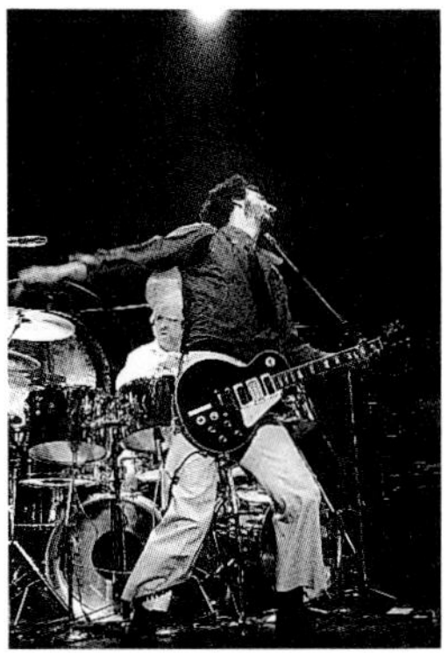

Nevertheless, when I look at the pictures, I think that this was the worst session I have ever done. And why? Because I realised I am still intimidated by Pete Townshend, by The Who and what they all stood for - to me.

In retrospect, I should have told him to fuck off and not bother. But what did I do? I asked him for an autograph.

I'm still a fan.

Ross Halfin

Keith Moon, '78

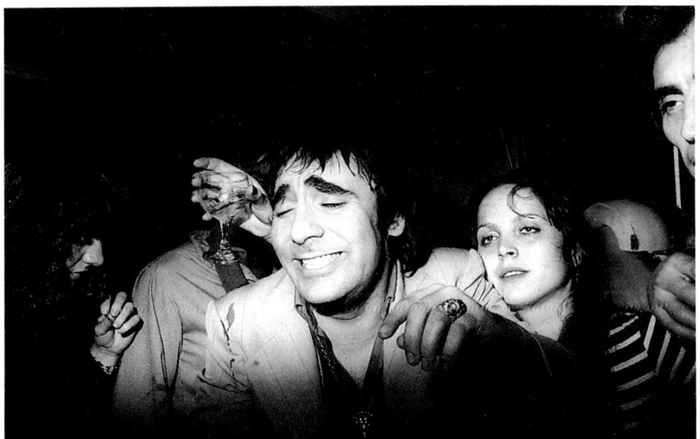

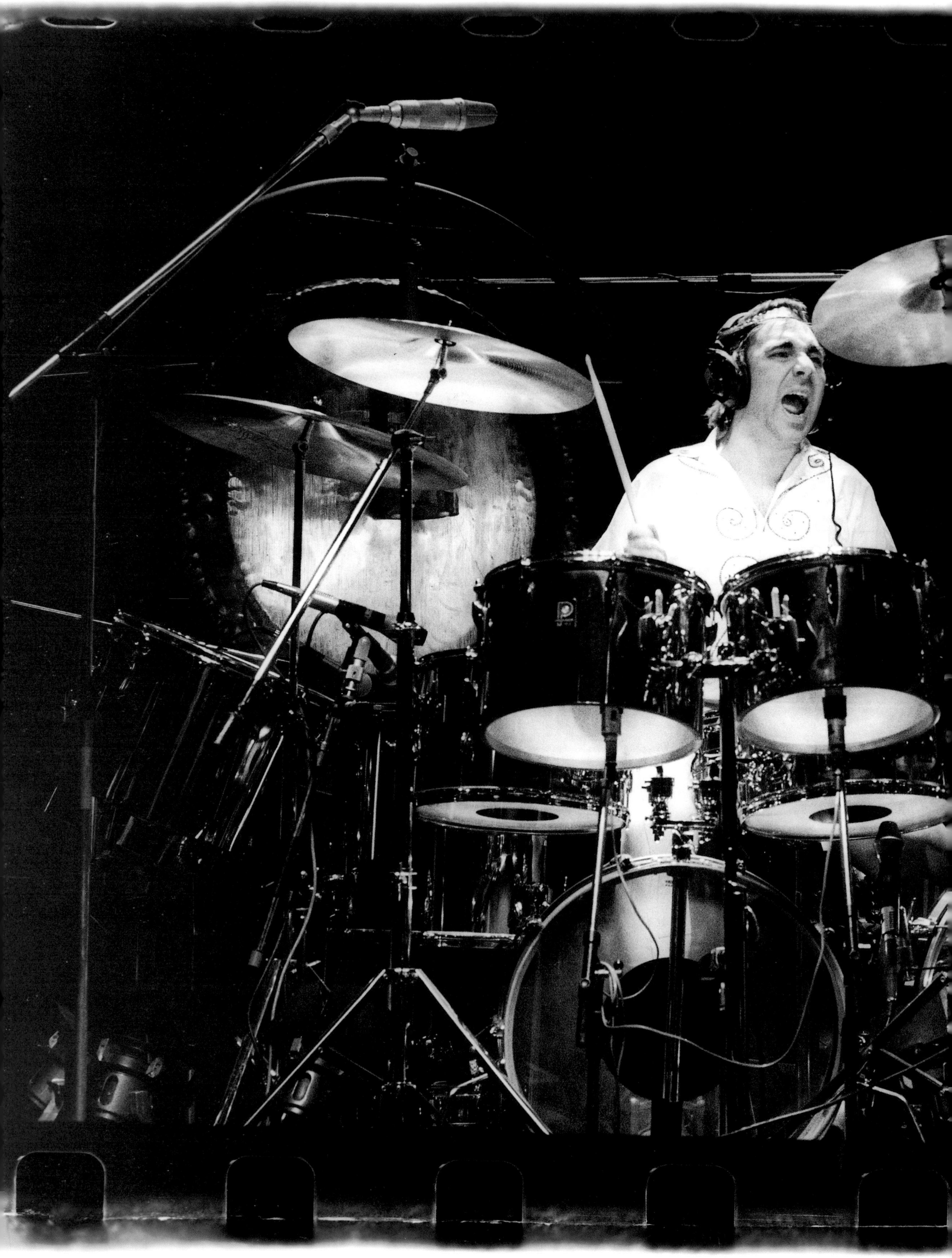

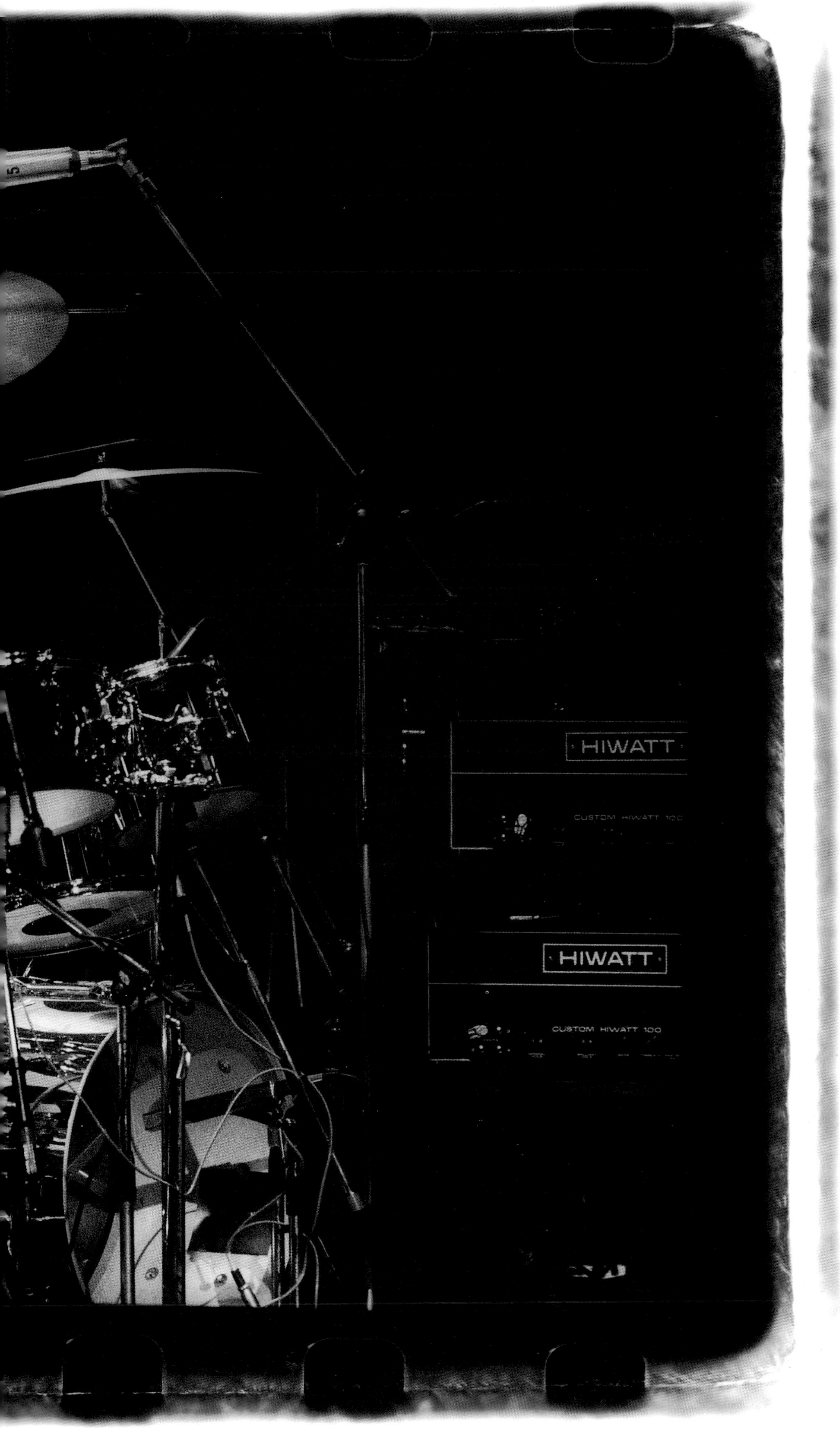

Keith Moon's
Last Gig,
Shepperton
May 25, 1978

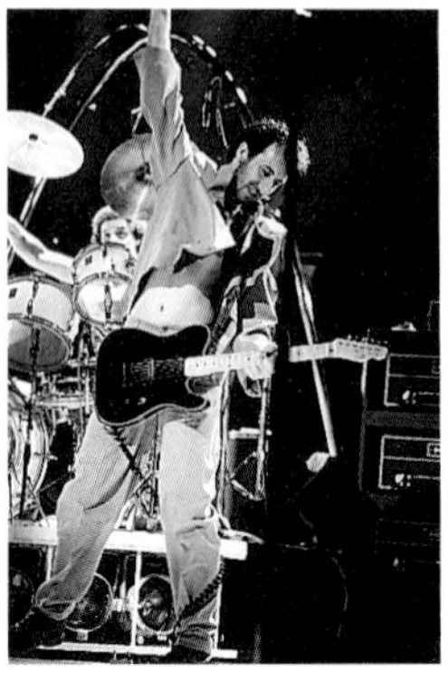
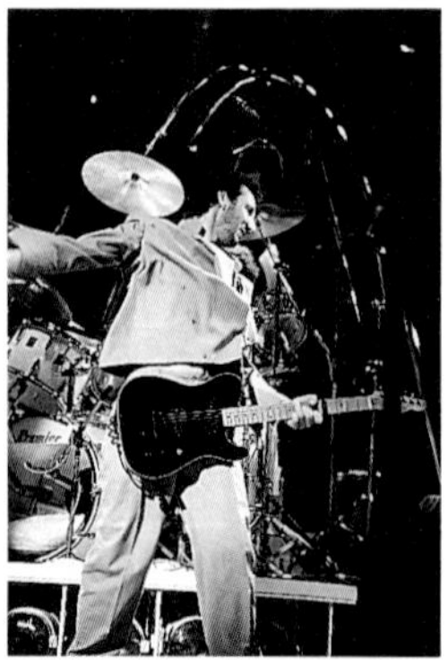
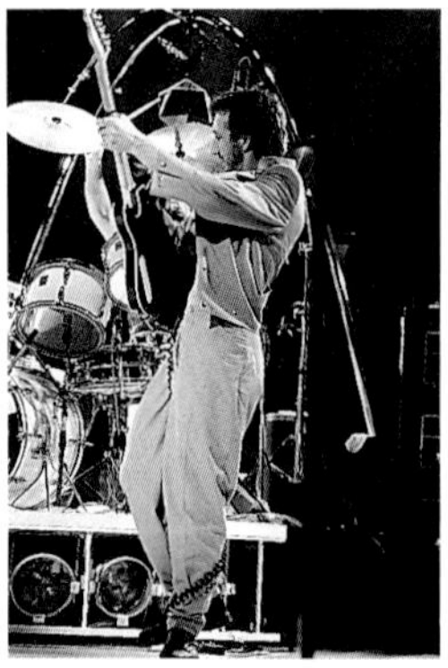
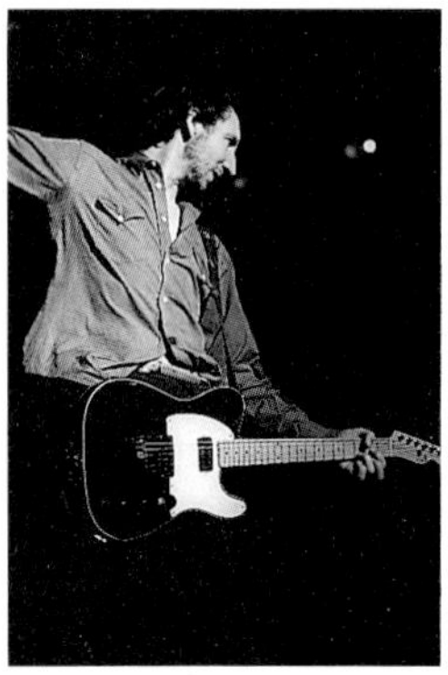
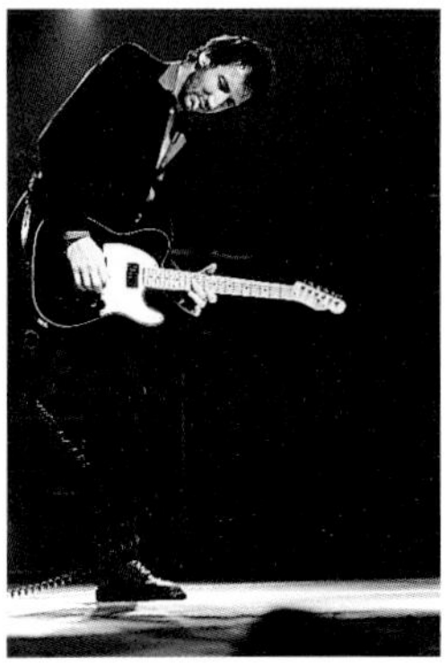
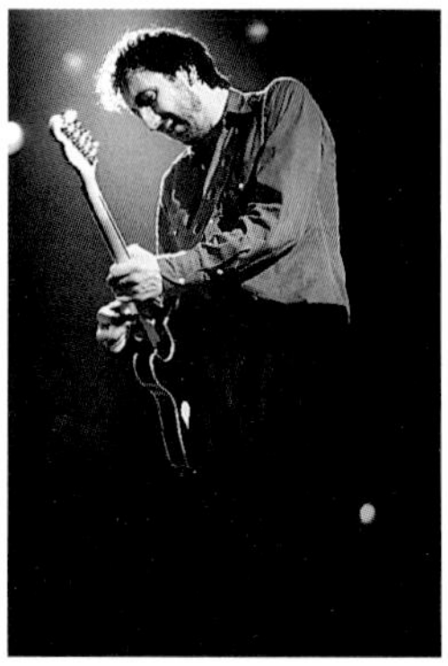
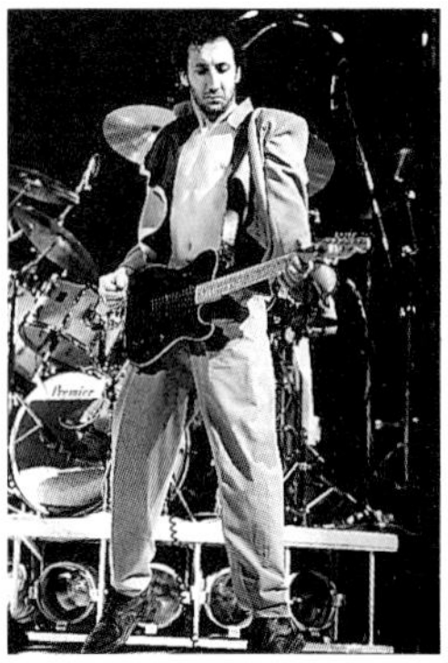
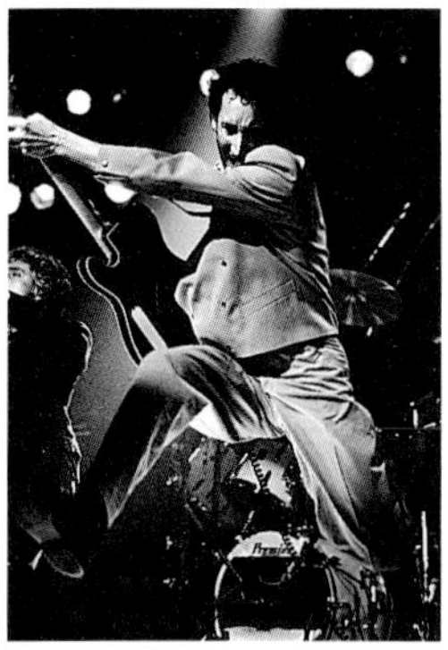
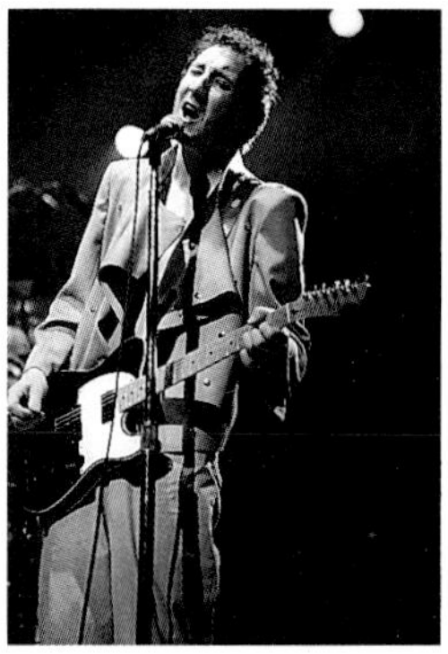
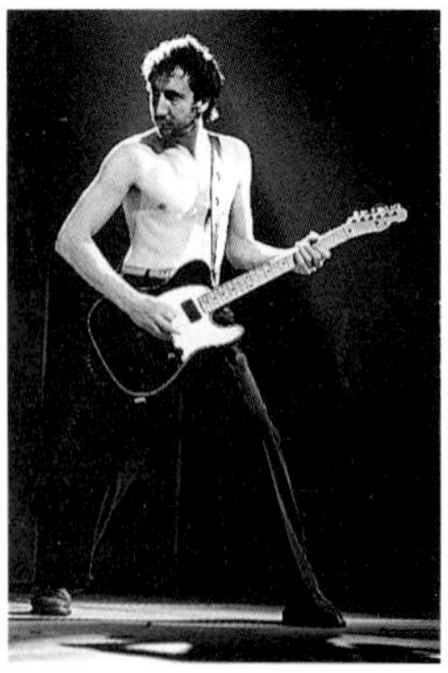
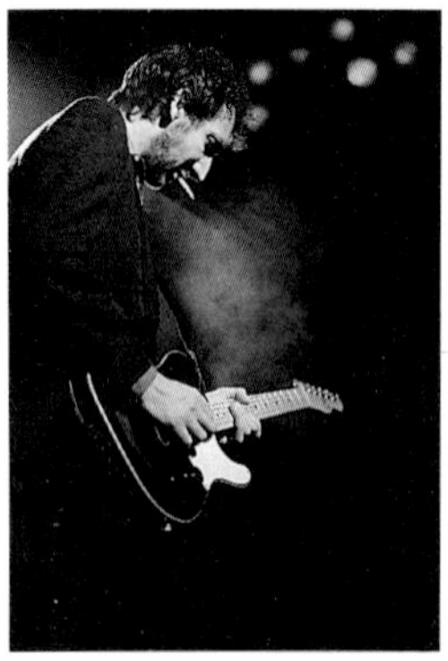
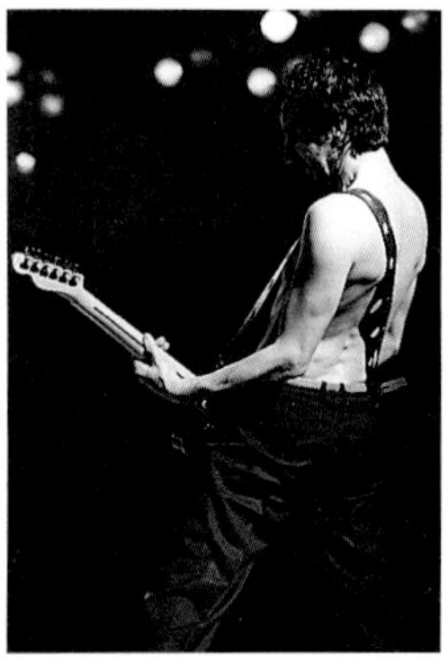

Pete Townshend
"Under The Influence"
Rainbow Theatre,
February 3 & 4, 1981
"The Most Self-Indulgent Who Shows I Ever Saw."

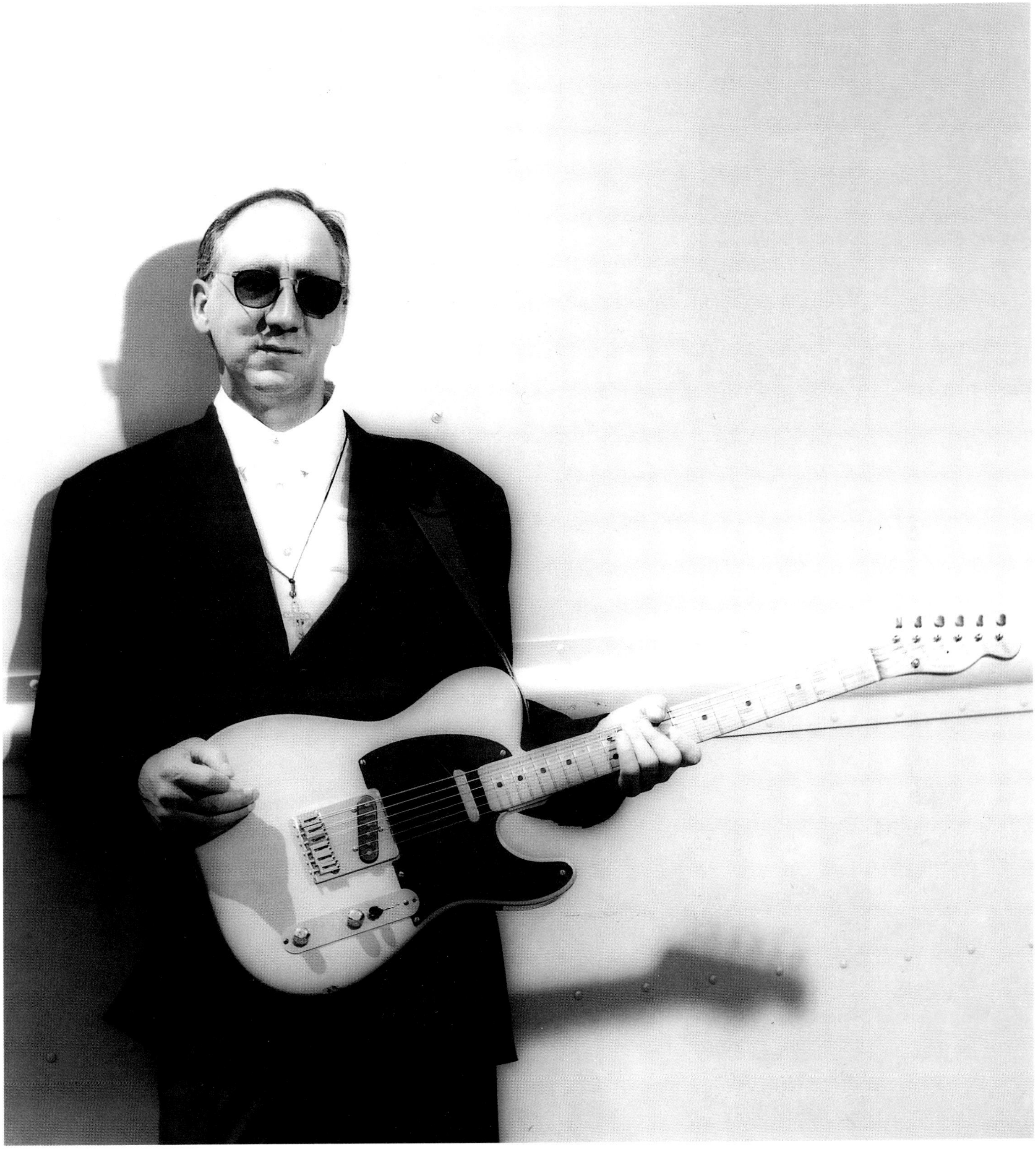

Pete Townshend
Burbank, July '93

eddie vedder

Eddie Vedder
Berkeley '93

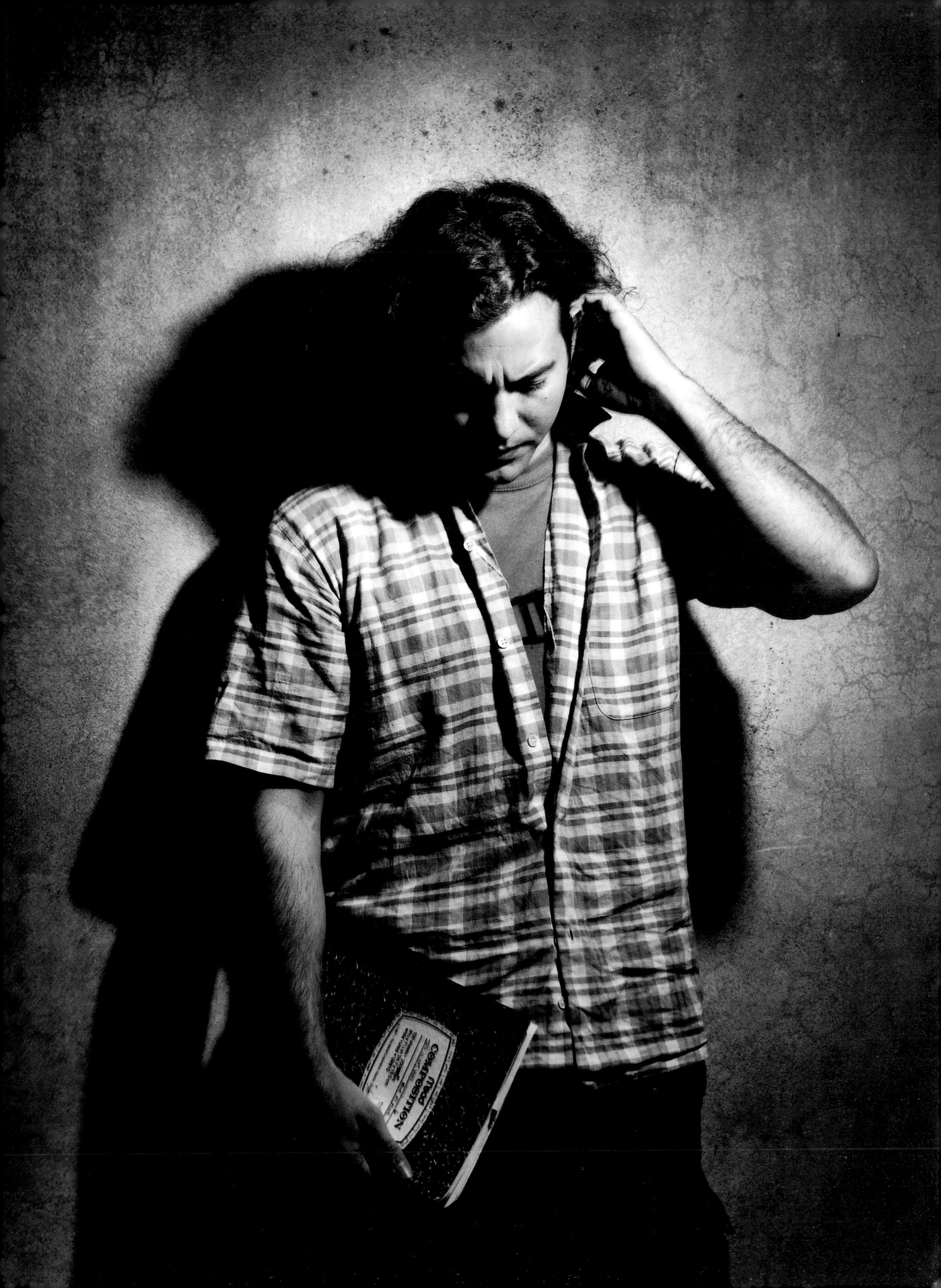
Mead
COMPOSITION

EDDIE VEDDER

I was in San Jose in the summer of 1993 working the Rollins Band, who were touring at that time with Pearl Jam. While I was there, I took the opportunity to ask Eddie Vedder - a major Who fan - if he'd fancy writing something on Pete Townshend for the book and - very kind man that he is - he said yes.

The last time I saw Eddie was the next day at the Greek Theater in San Francisco, and I asked him how his essay was coming along. And he said, "I'm a bit behind, actually. My head's in the right place, but I'm a bit late with my paper."

I'm still waiting on him.

ROSS HALFIN

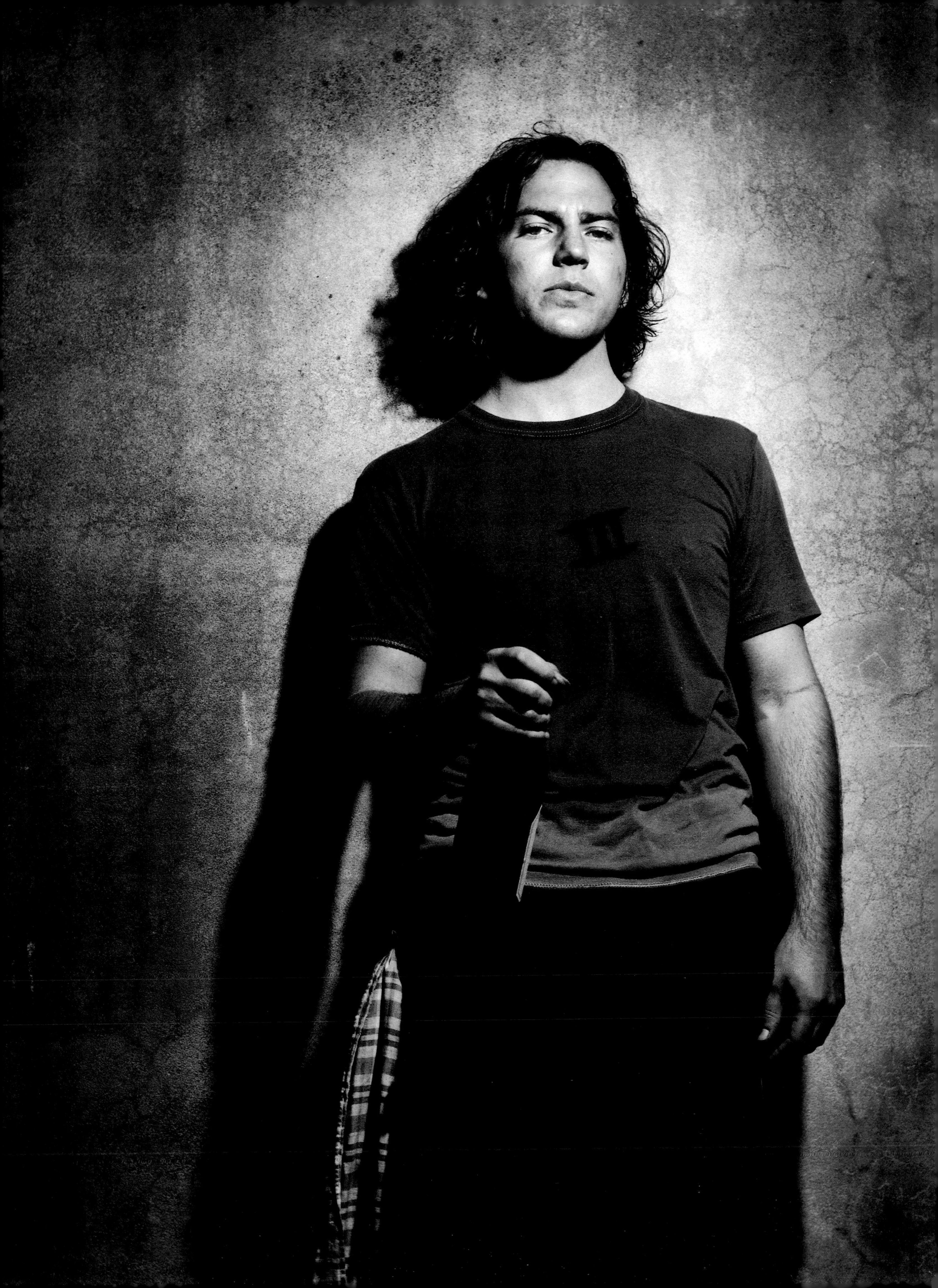

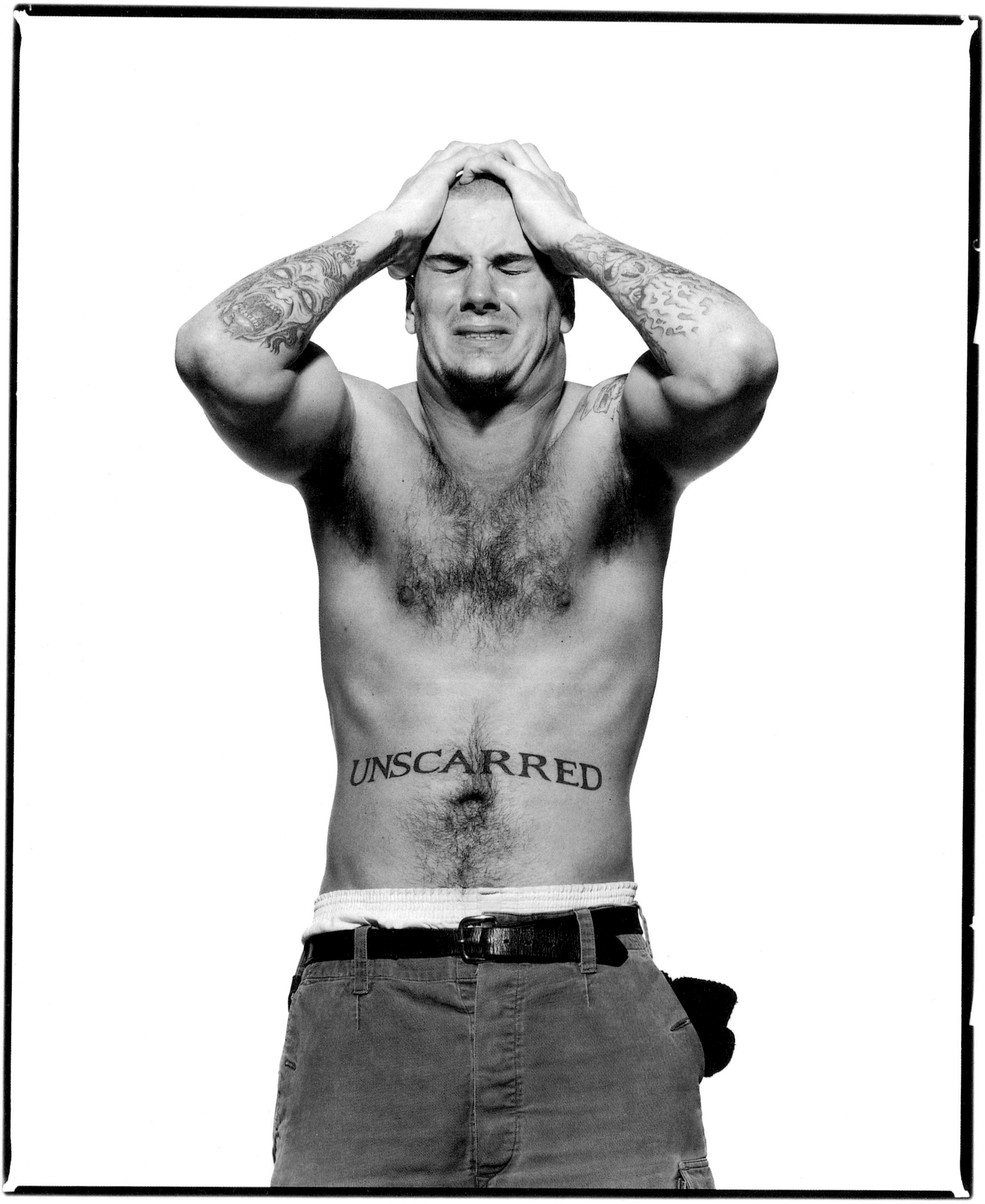
UNSCARRED

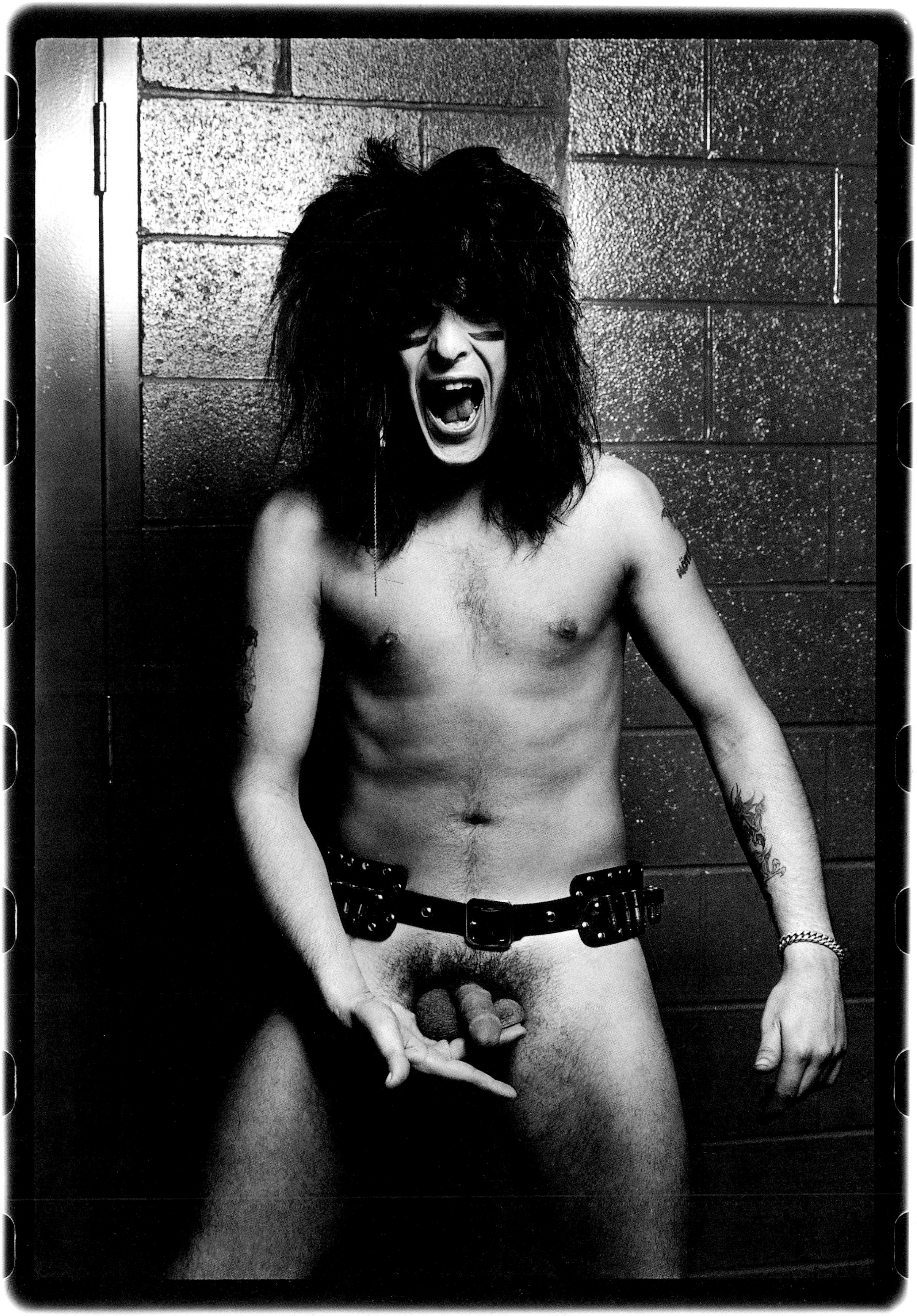

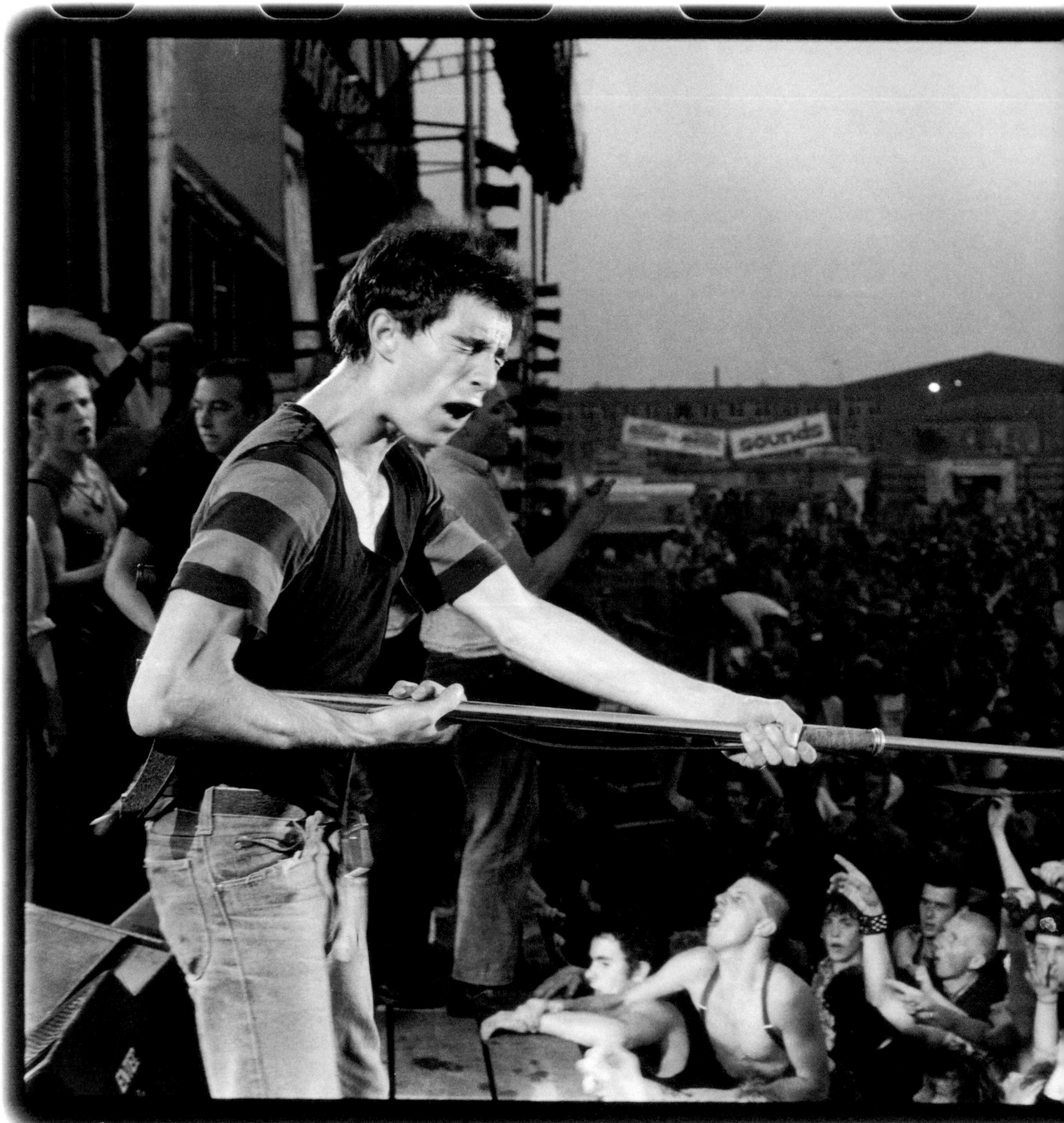
sounds

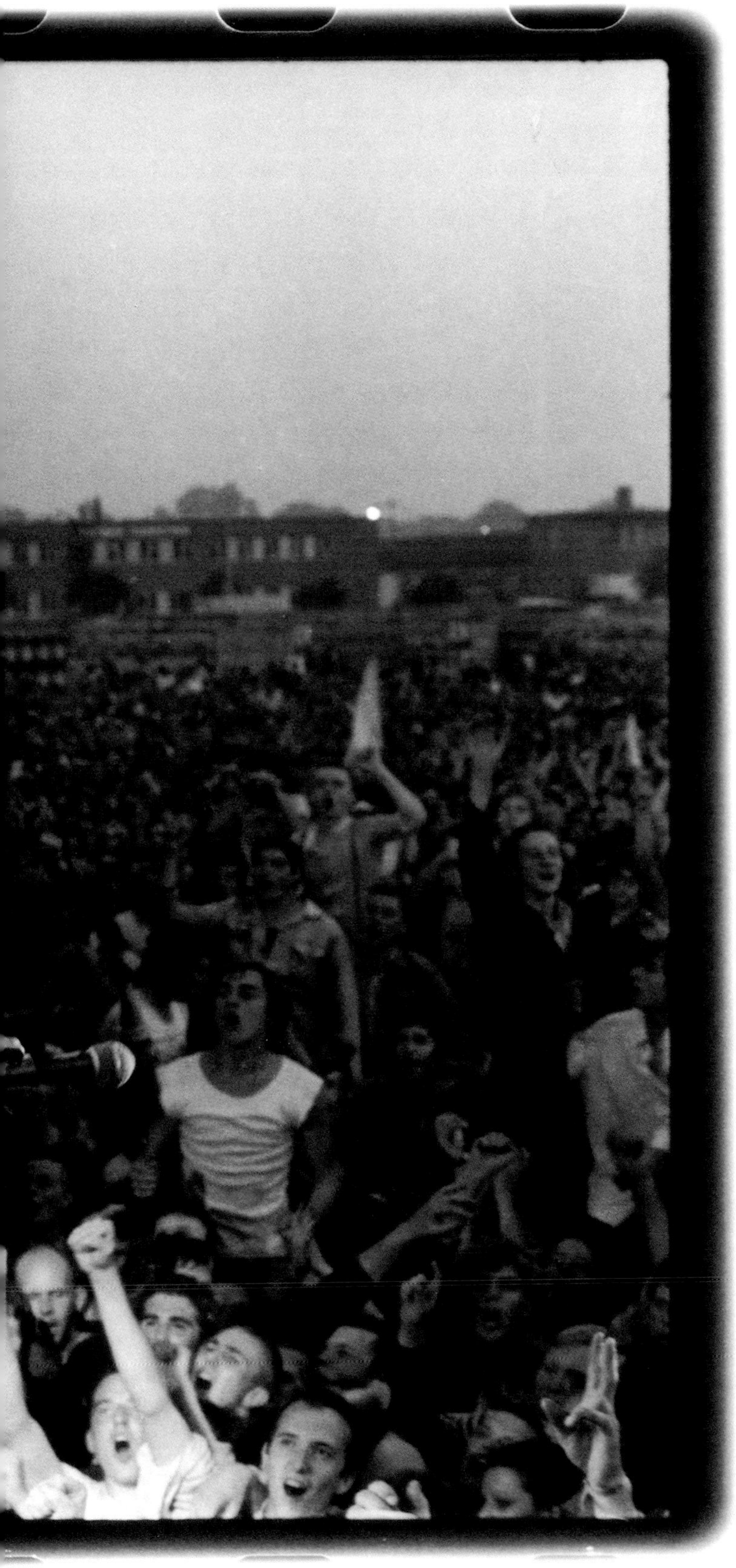

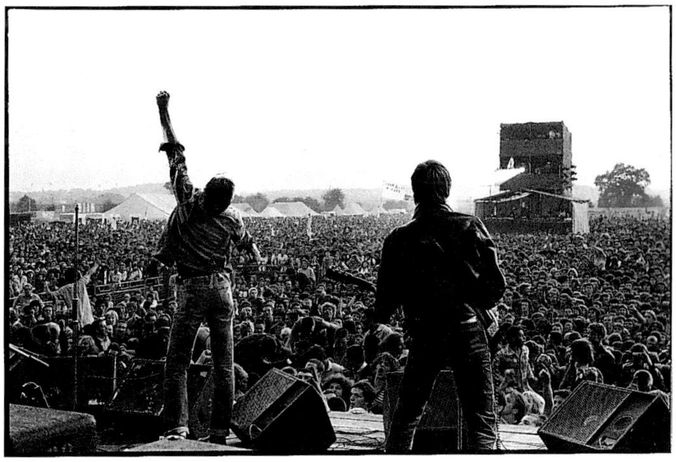

SHAM 69

"They brought a skinhead entourage who terrorised and fought the audience. They were pathetic."

–Ross Halfin

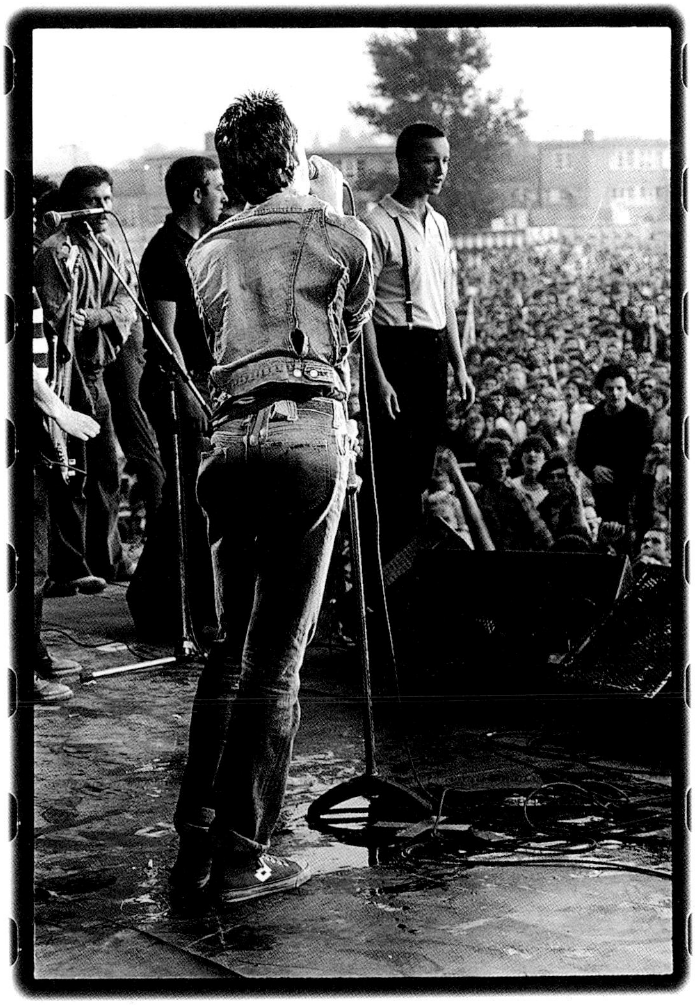

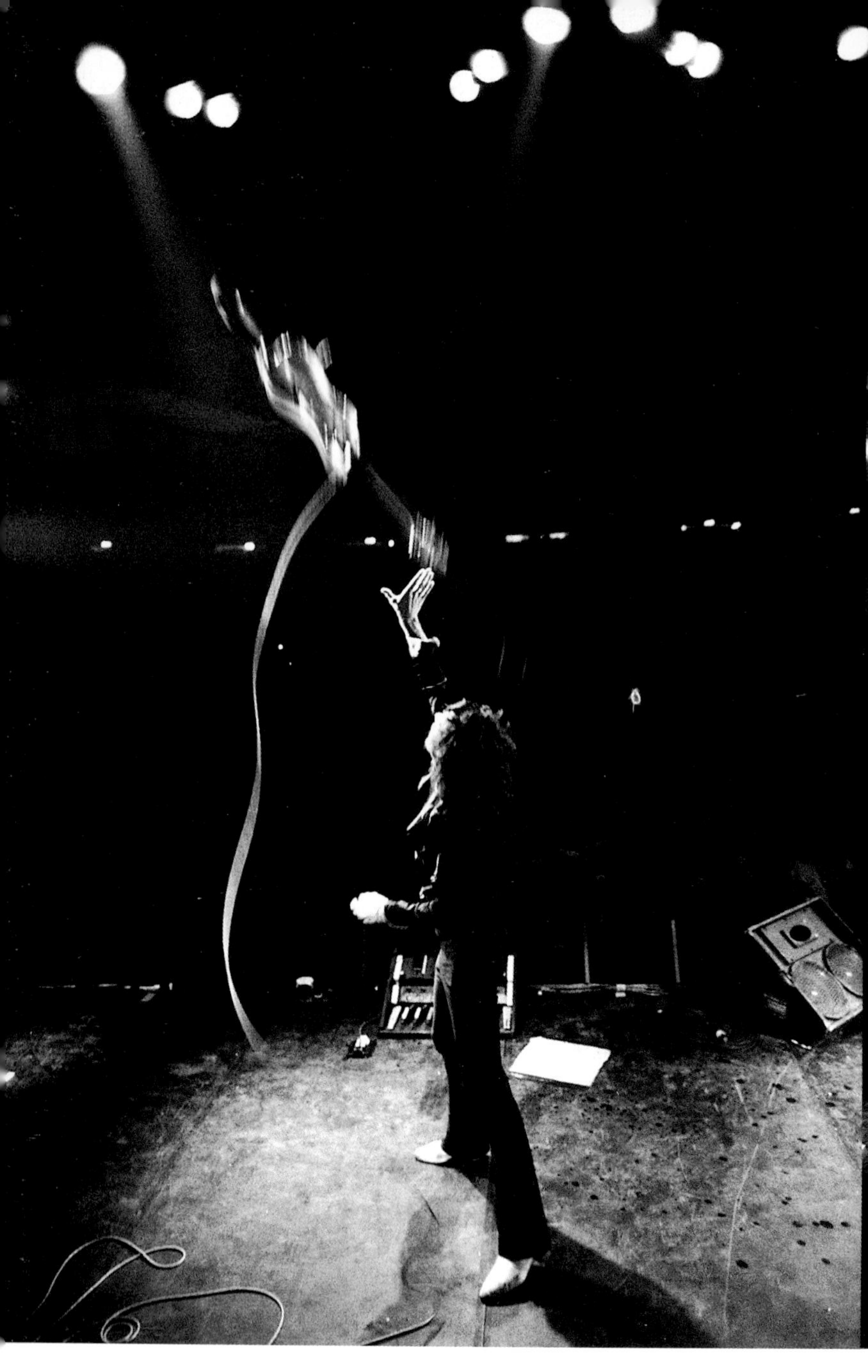

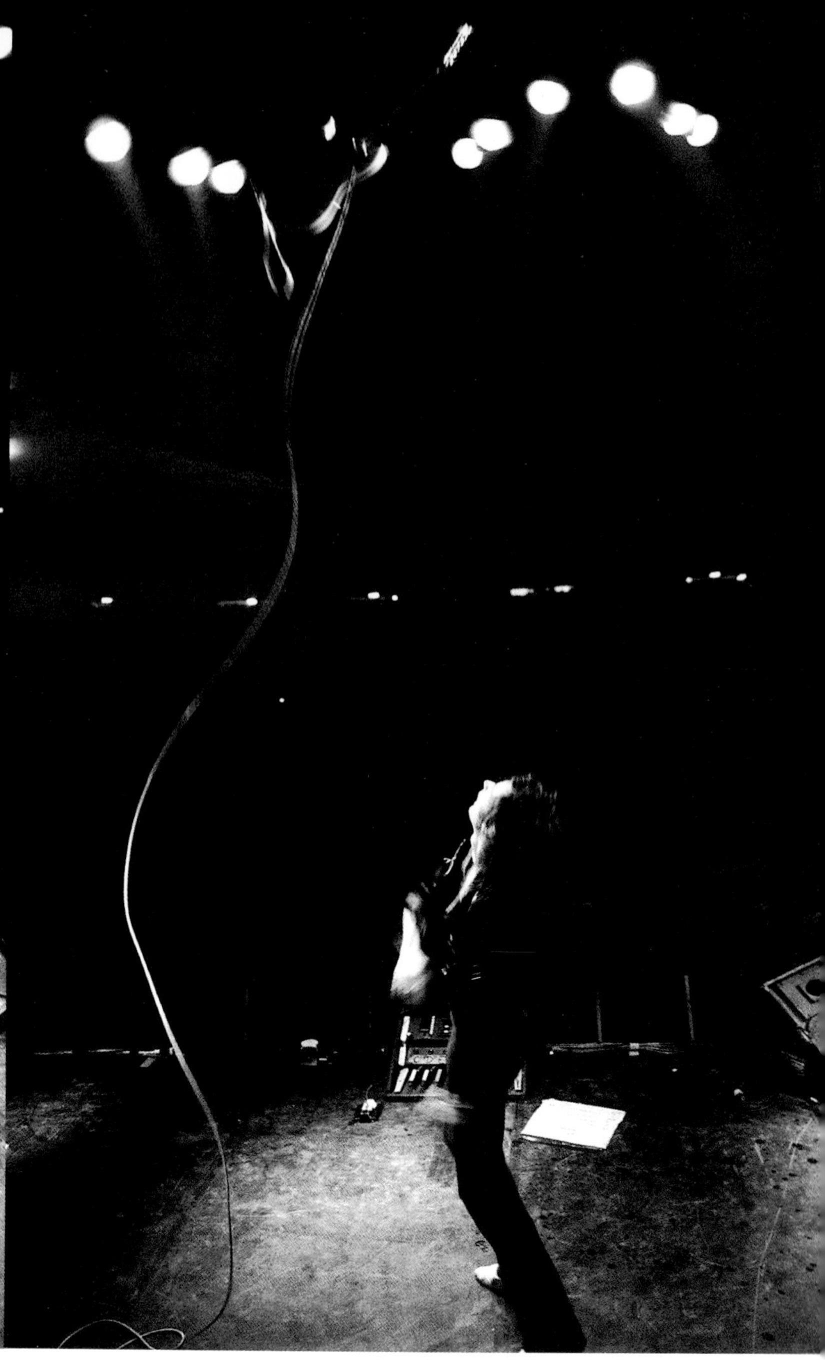

RITCHIE BLACKMORE

THE BASTARD IN BLACK

Mean, Moody, Arrogant, Self Obsessed, Selfish, Insecure, Bitter. . . . . Ritchie Blackmore posesses all these character defects. Get on his dark side and a worse enemy would be hard to find (ask anyone he's fired).

A Total Bastard. . . . .

In the early seventies, Deep Purple were one of the world's leading purveyors of a symphonic heavy metal sound that is still synonymous in the world of rock. Blackmore's distinctive distorted tremelo sound has been copied many times along with his sombre "lone wolf outlaw" image.

I met the man when still in my early teens and we hit it off as we had many things in common: Mandrax, Johnny Walker Black Label, strong German beer and the intense love of large breasts. The man was also my fuckin' hero and having him as a friend was a dream come true.

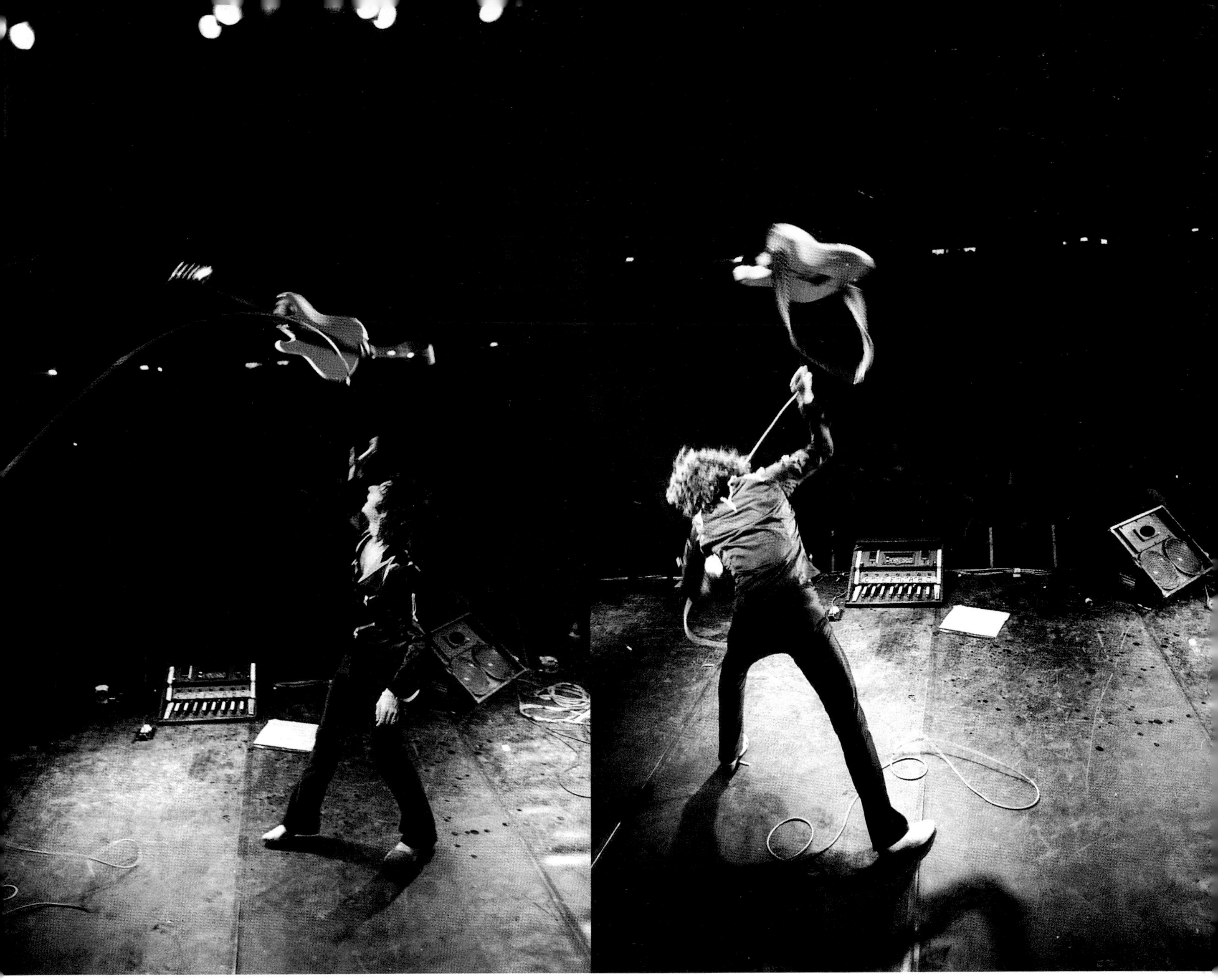

Ritchie Blackmore, Europe '80

Onstage, I have seen him at his best; offstage I've witnessed the tantrums. But for all his shitty qualities, I still really like the man, he's real.

Nowadays Deep Purple are no longer a force to be reckoned with; their sound is bloated, diluted and dated. It's been that way ever since Blackmore decided to take the AOR American Radio route. His influence is still felt today; there can't be too many self respecting guitar fans who don't recognize the opening chord sequence to "Smoke On The Water".

Blackmore has never received the critical acclaim he deserves. While his peers (Clapton, Beck, Page) enjoy the adulation and respect, the man in black remains in the shadows.

Pete Makowski

VICTORIA-VERSICHERUNG
Bendzko
BERLIN...

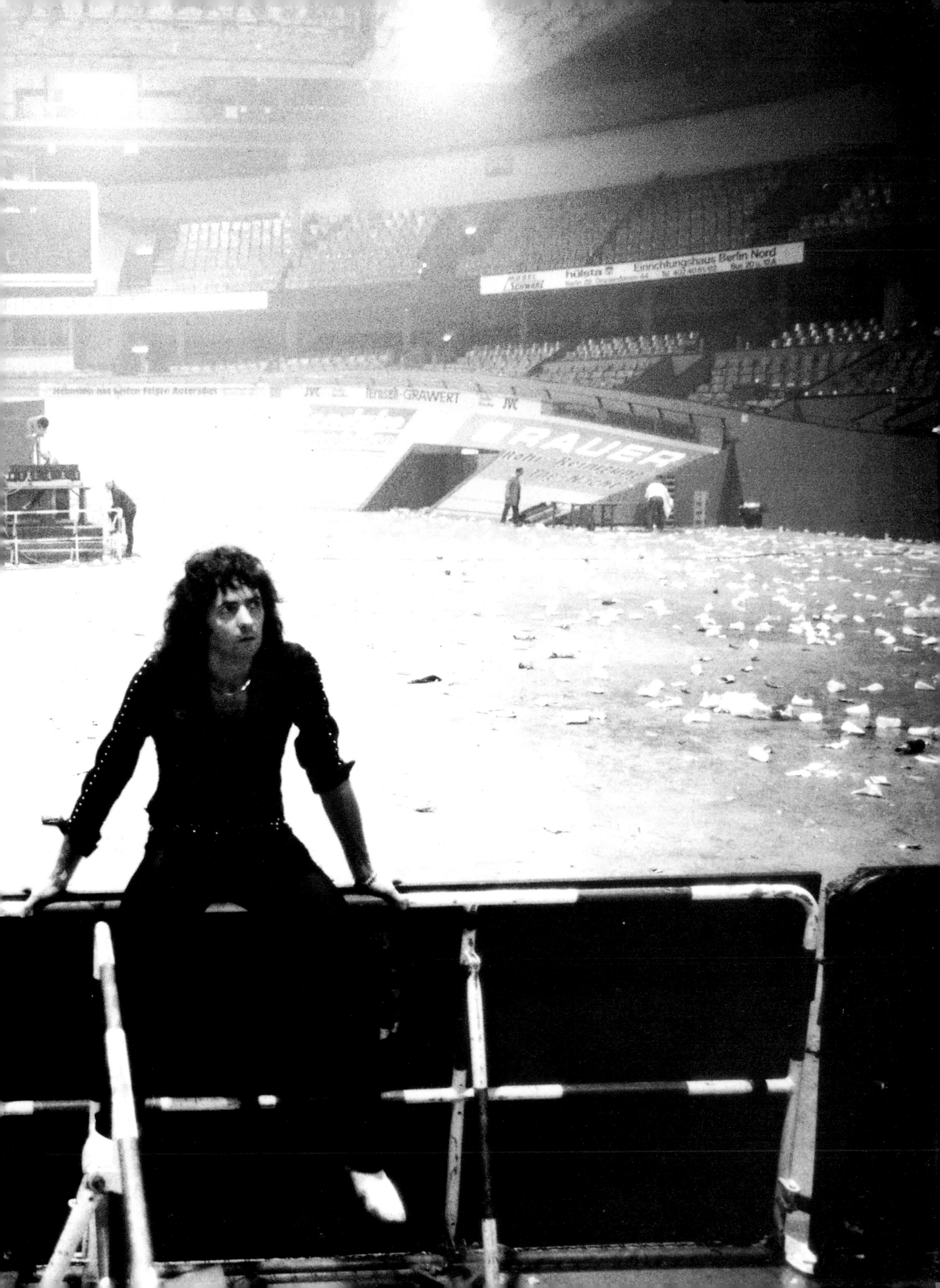
hülsta
Einrichtungshaus Berlin Nord
JVC
Fernseh-GRAWERT
JVC
BRAUER

page • plant

JIMMY PAGE & ROBERT PLANT
LAFAYETTE CEMETRY
NEW ORLEANS
MARCH 11, 1995

FOLLOWING PAGES:
PAGE/PLANT TOUR
1995

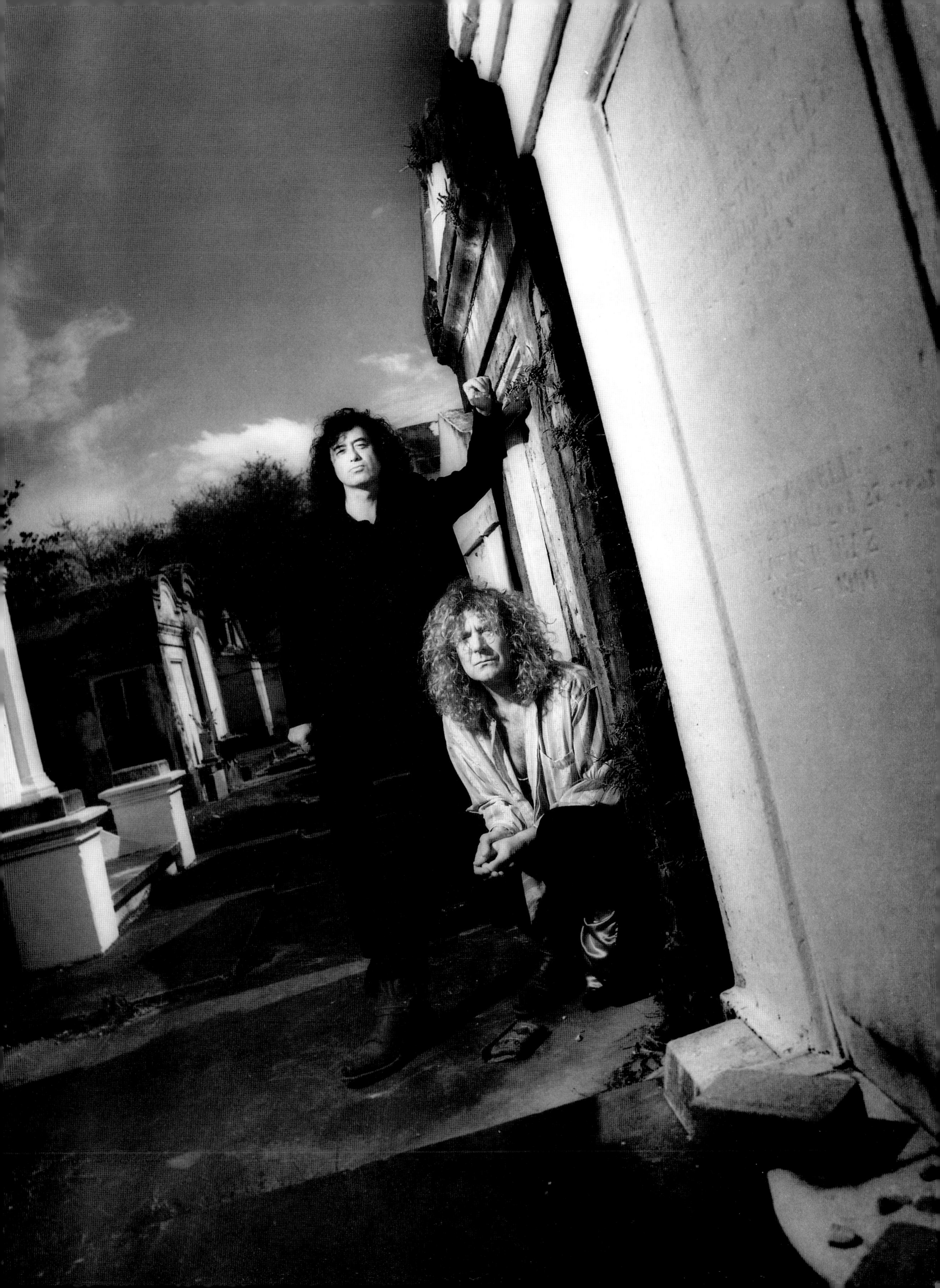

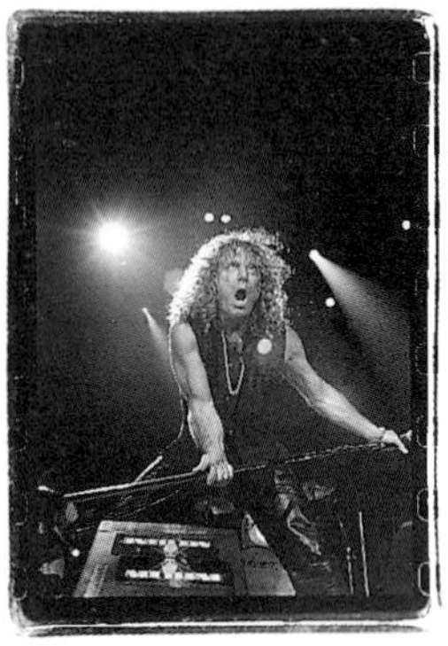
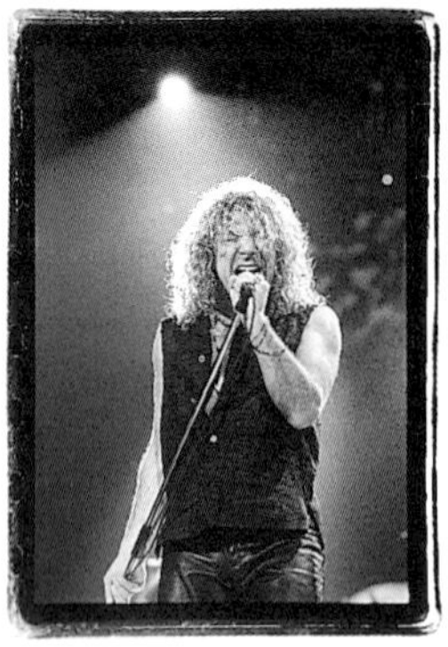
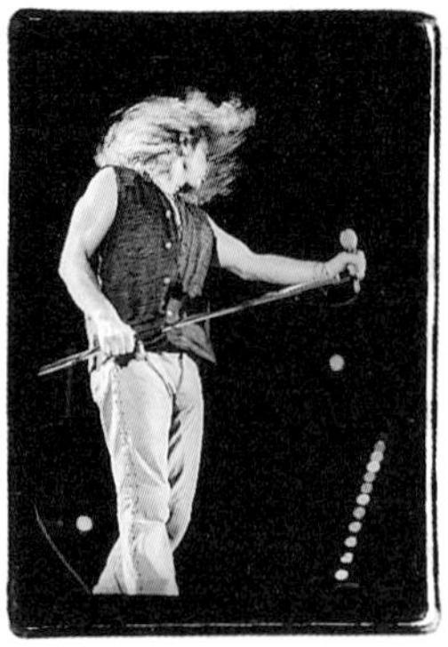
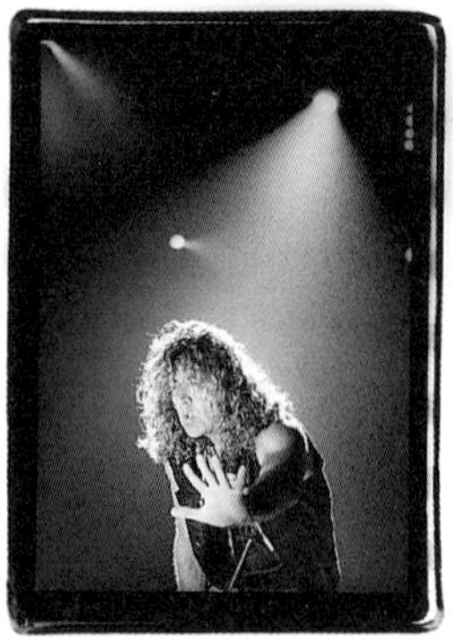
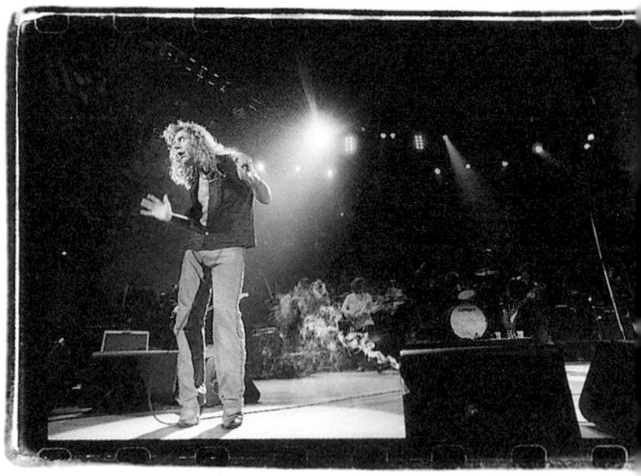
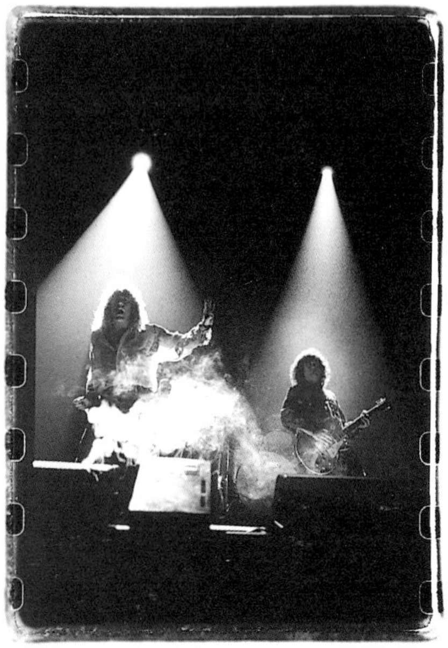
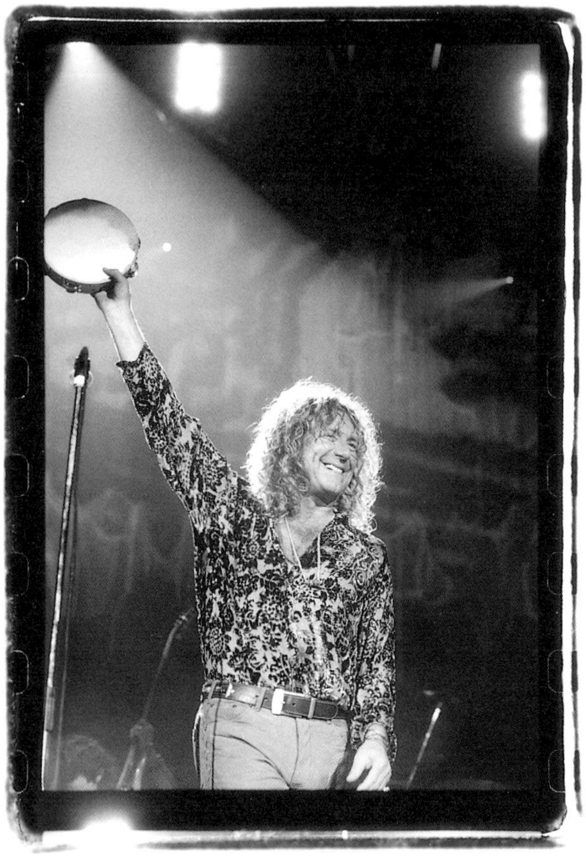
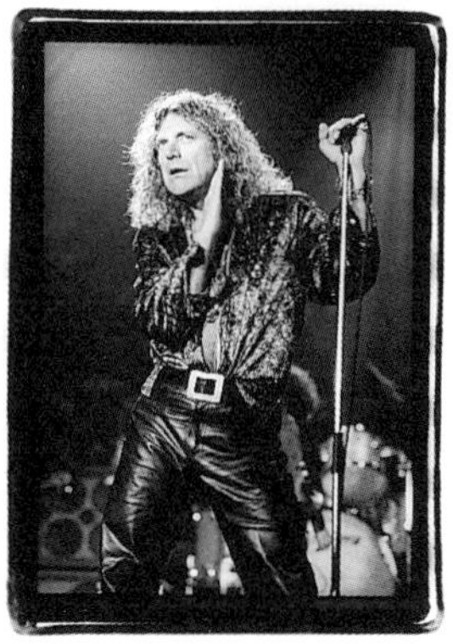
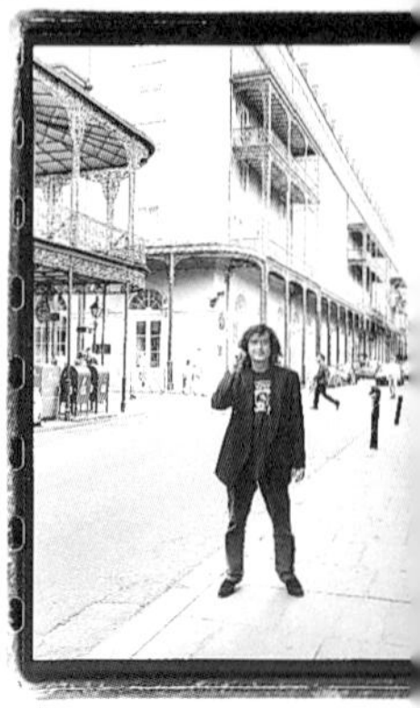
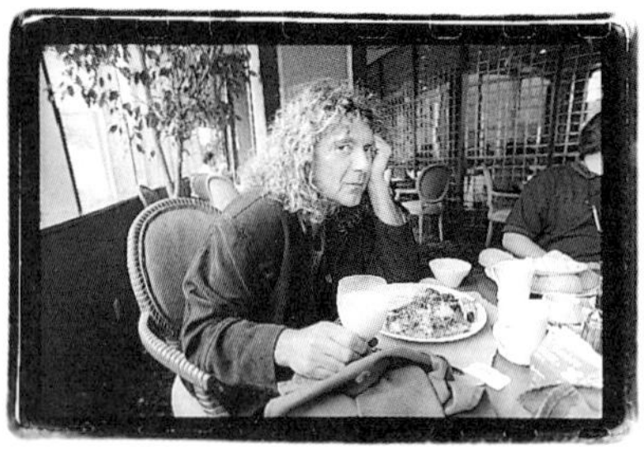
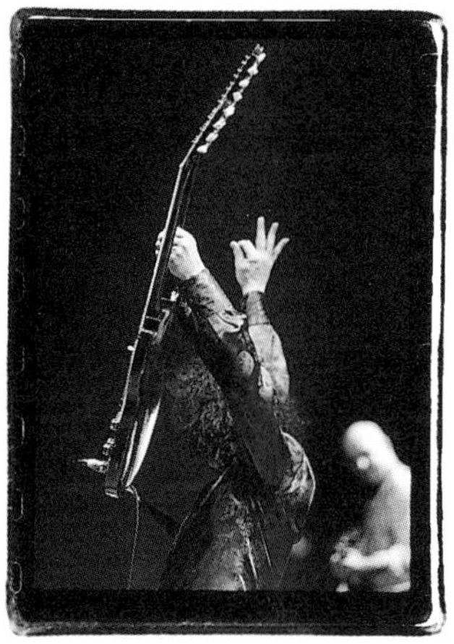
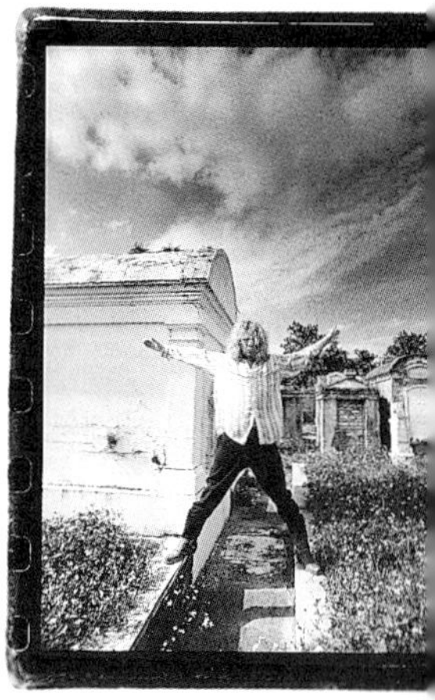
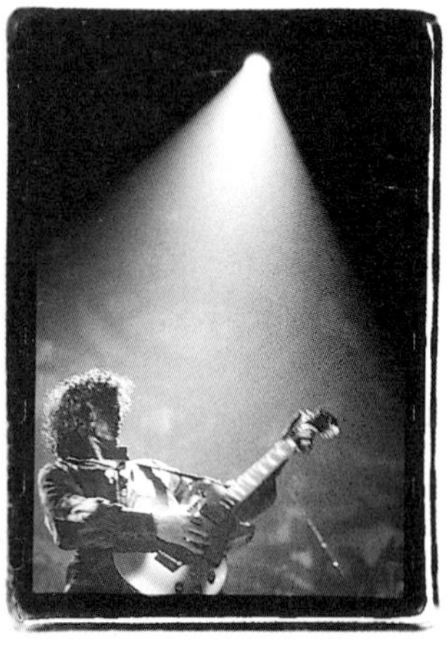
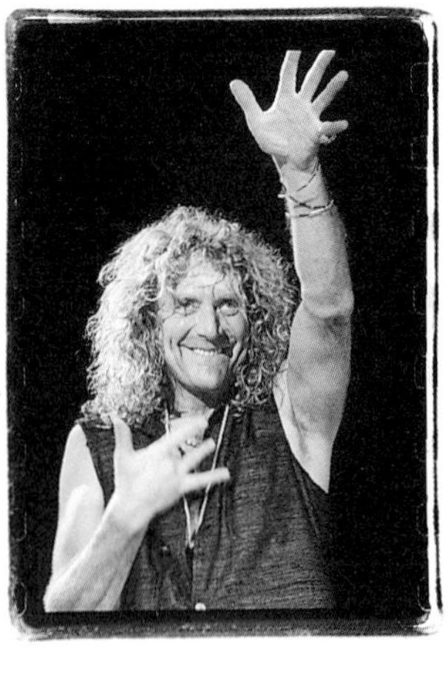
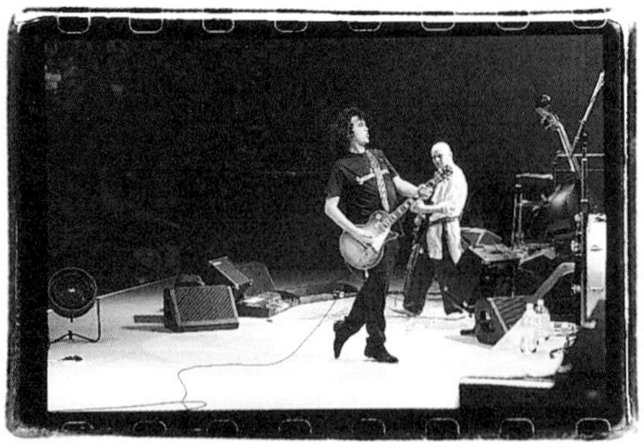
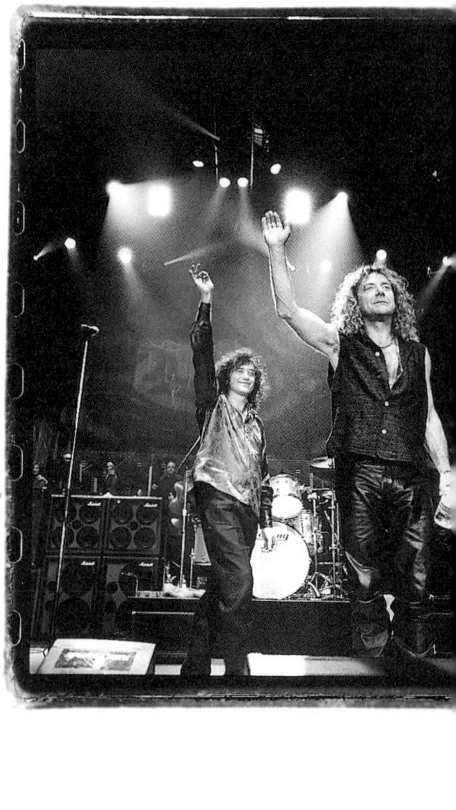
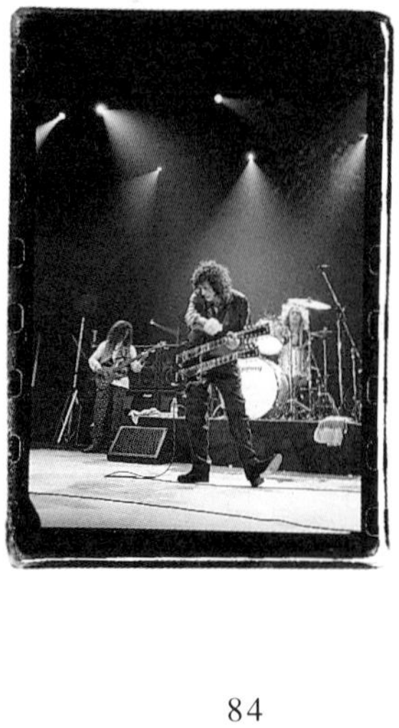
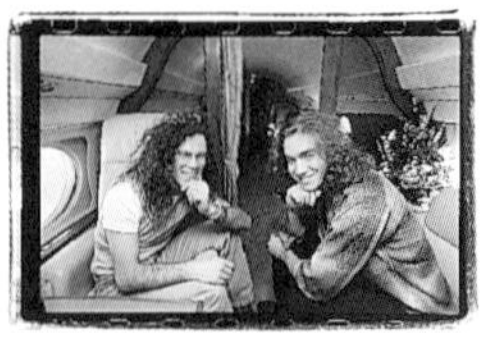
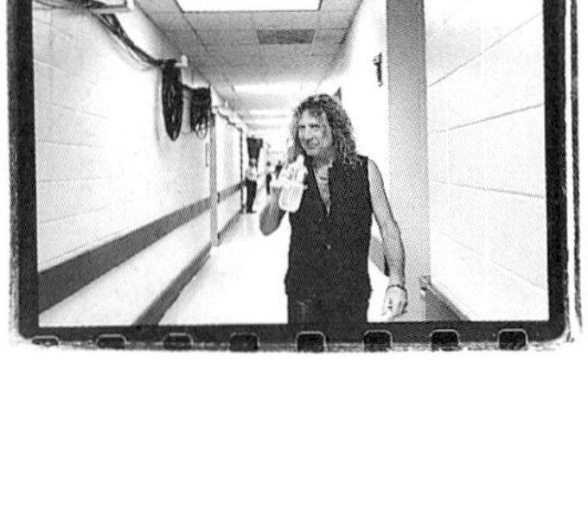
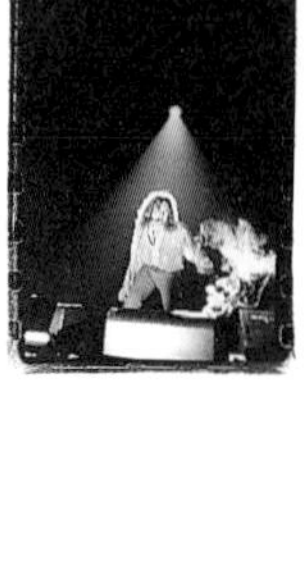
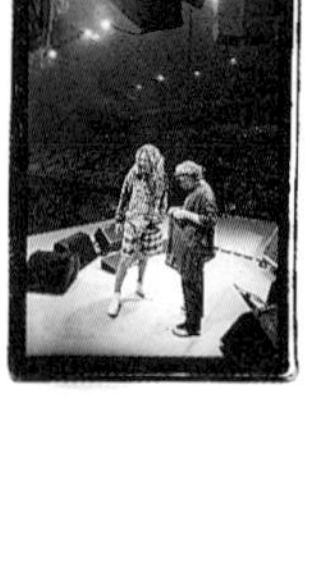
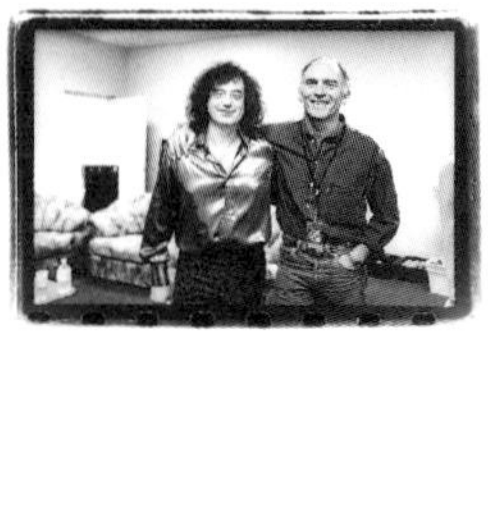

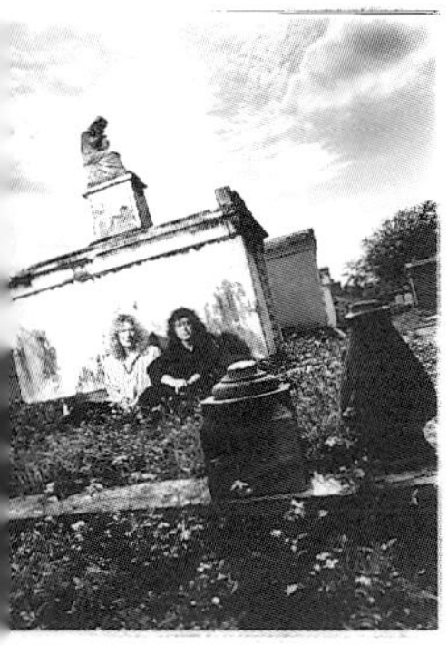
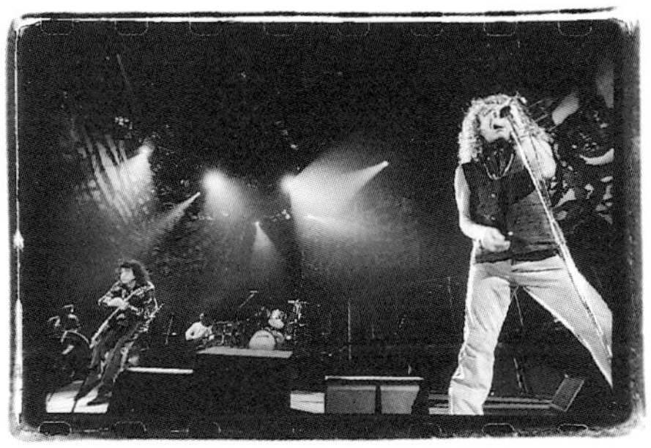
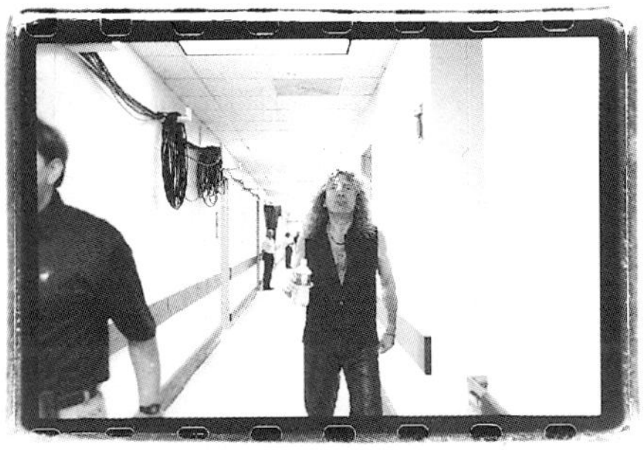
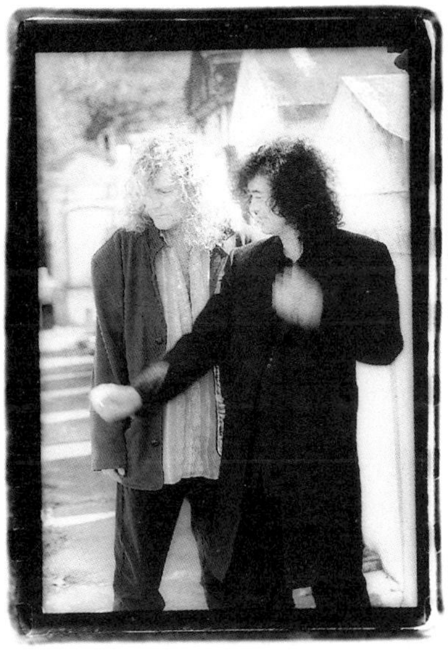
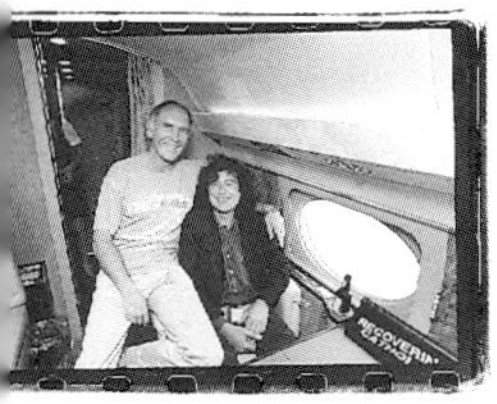
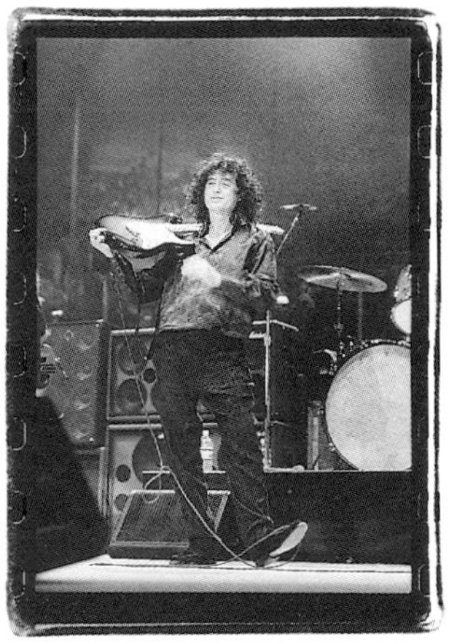
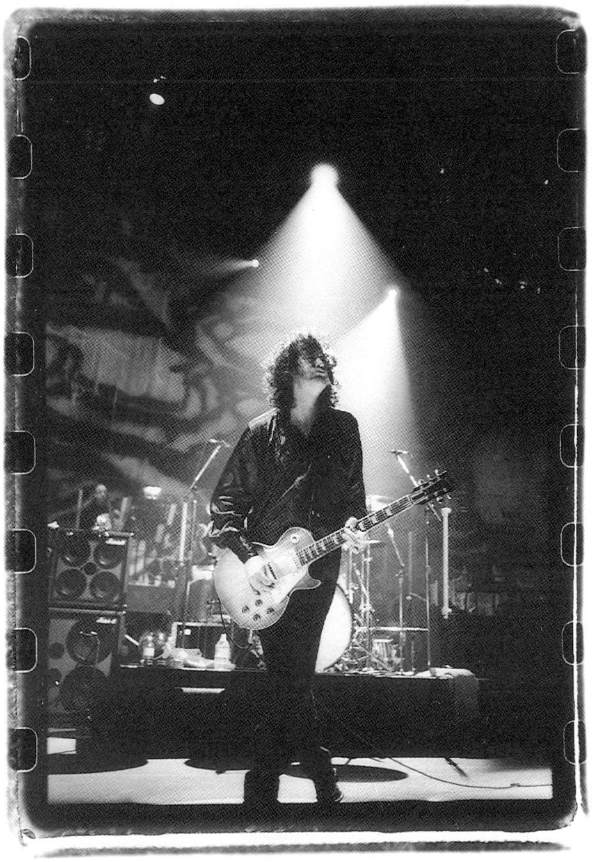
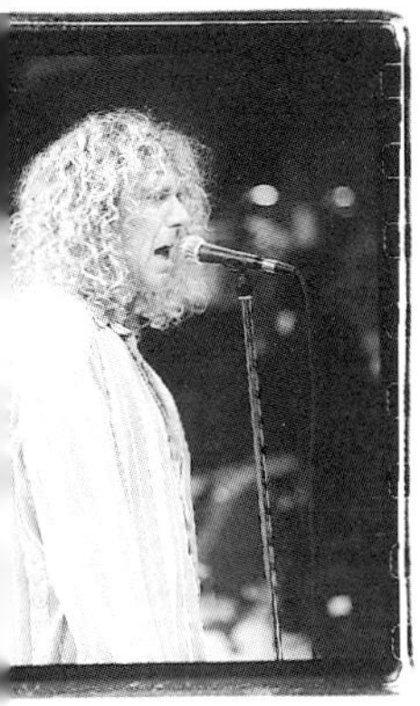
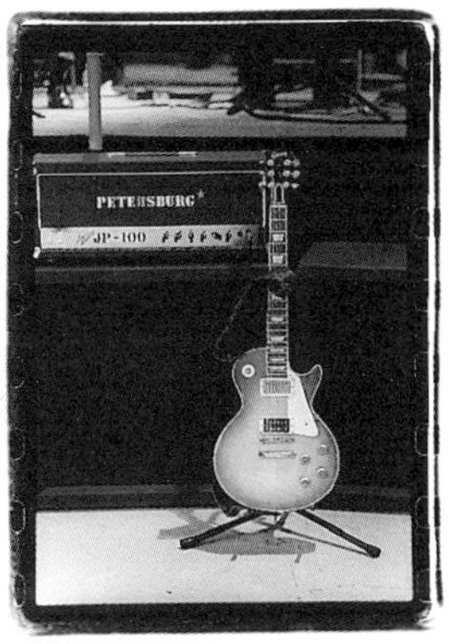
PETERSBURG
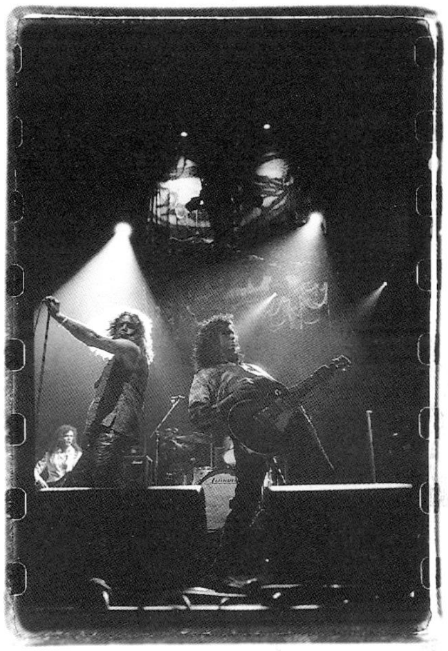
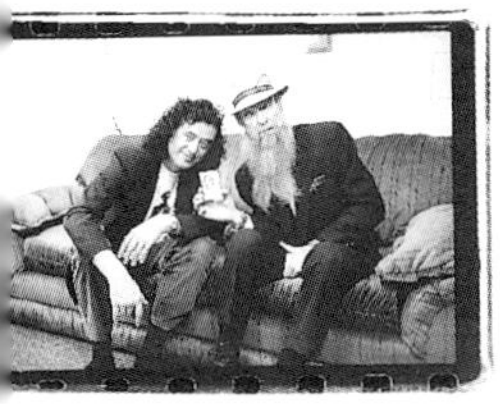
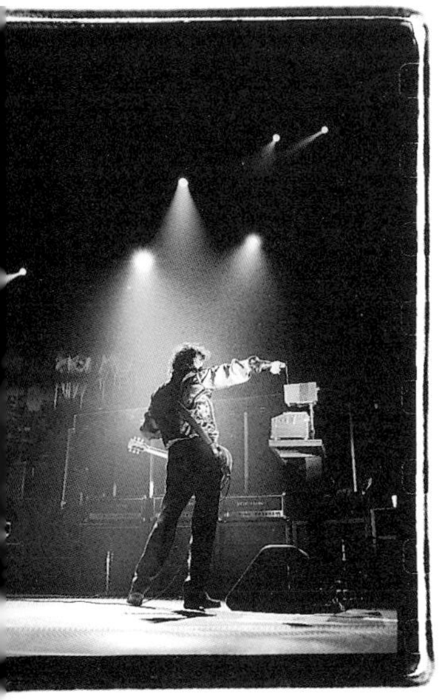
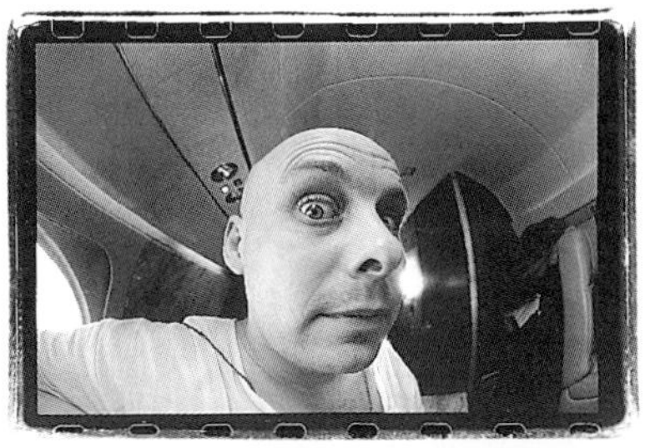
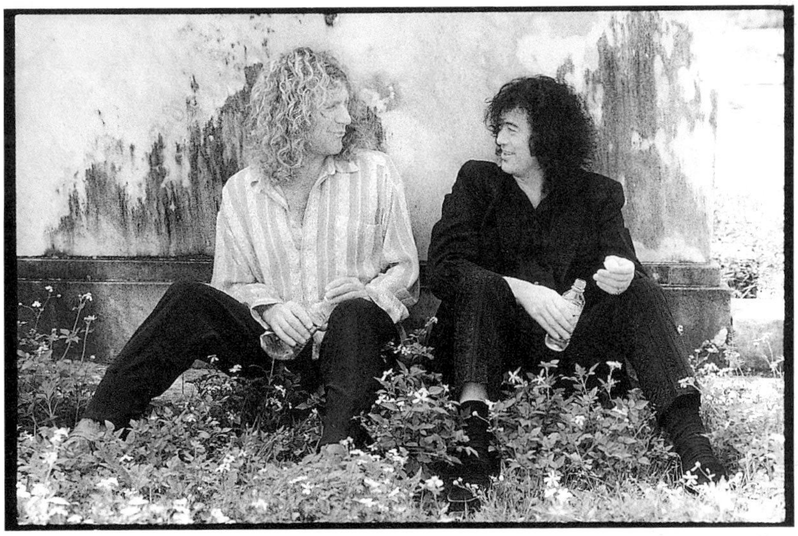
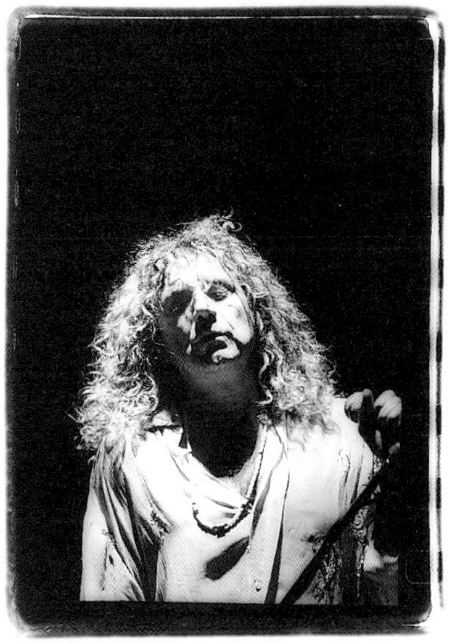
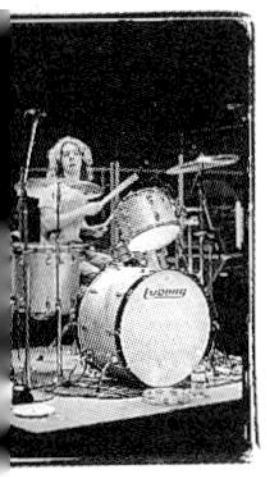
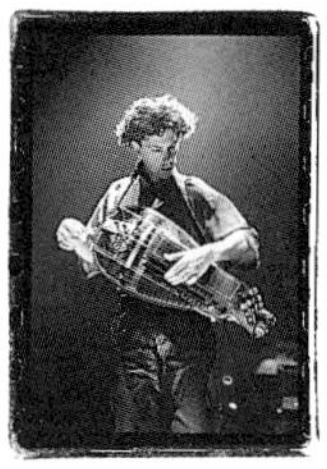
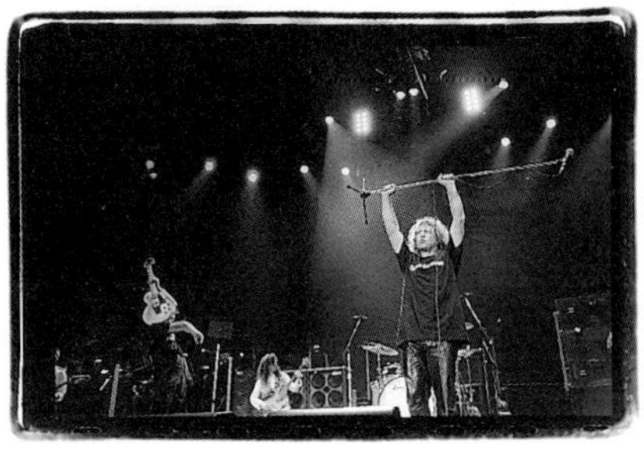
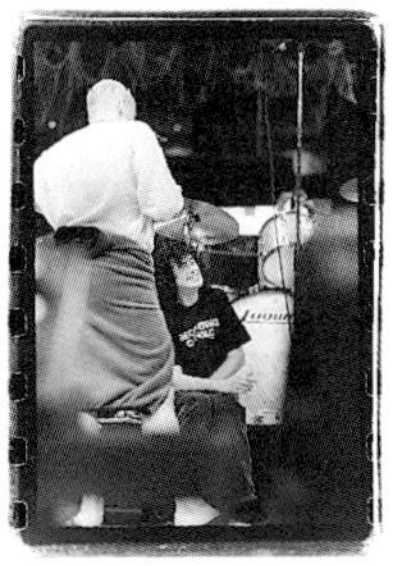
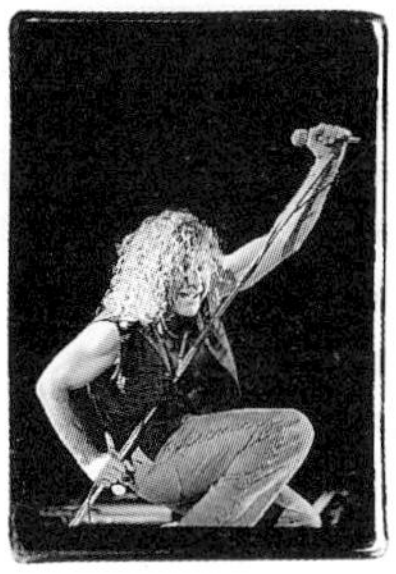

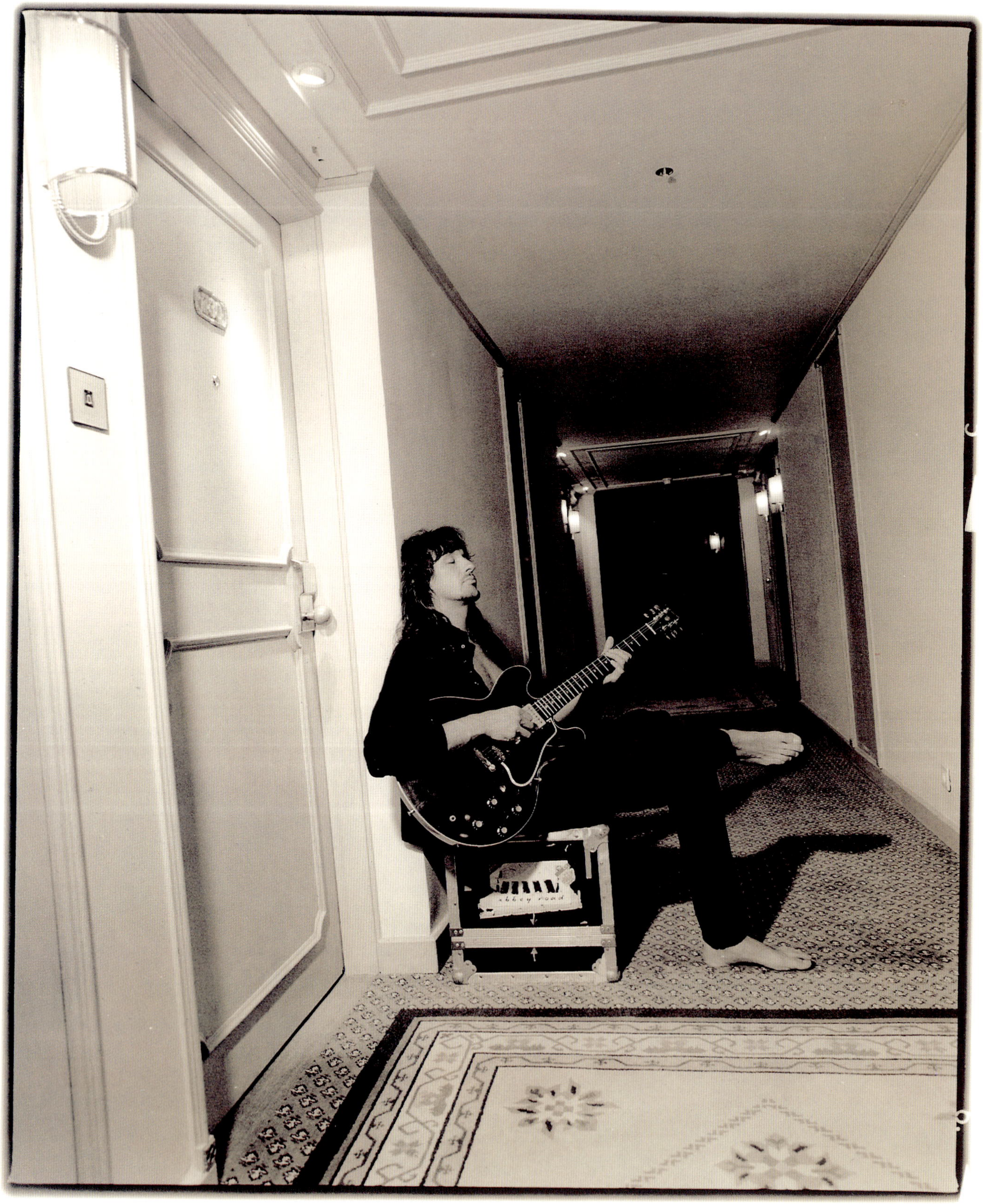

Richie Sambora
The Leela Kempinski
Bombay, '95

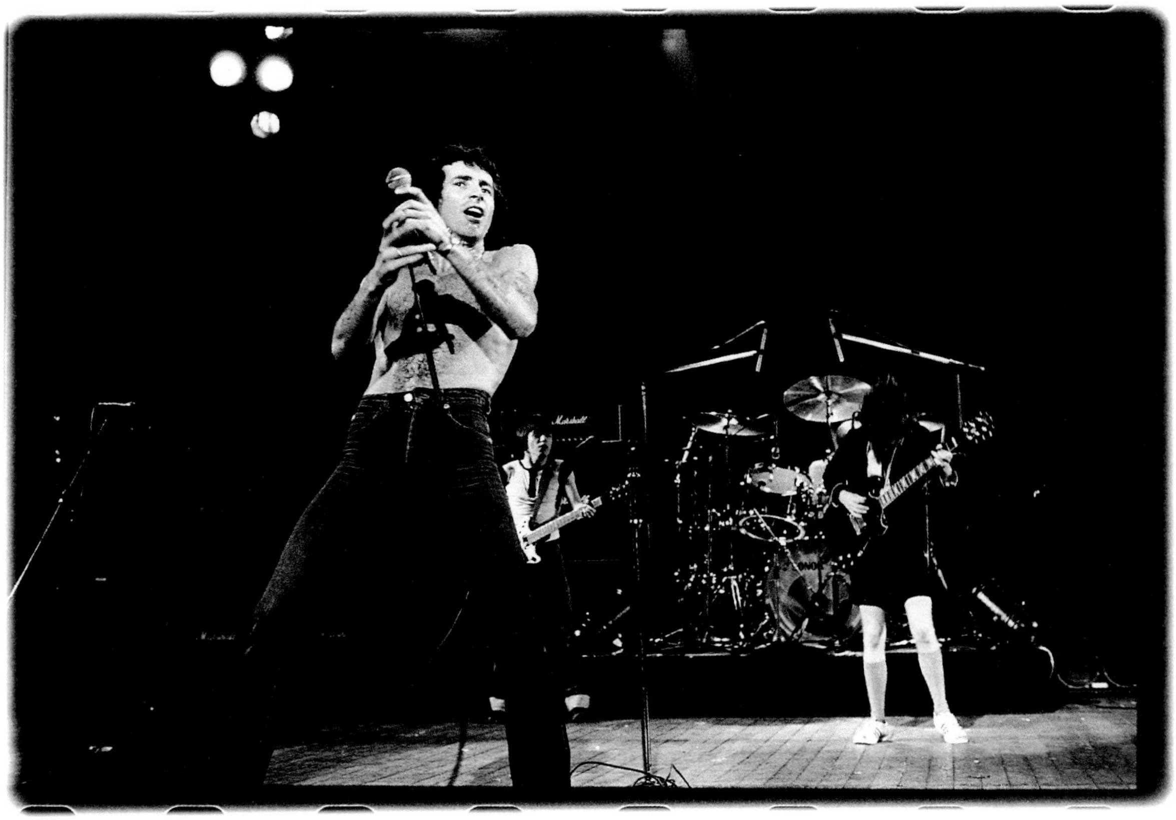

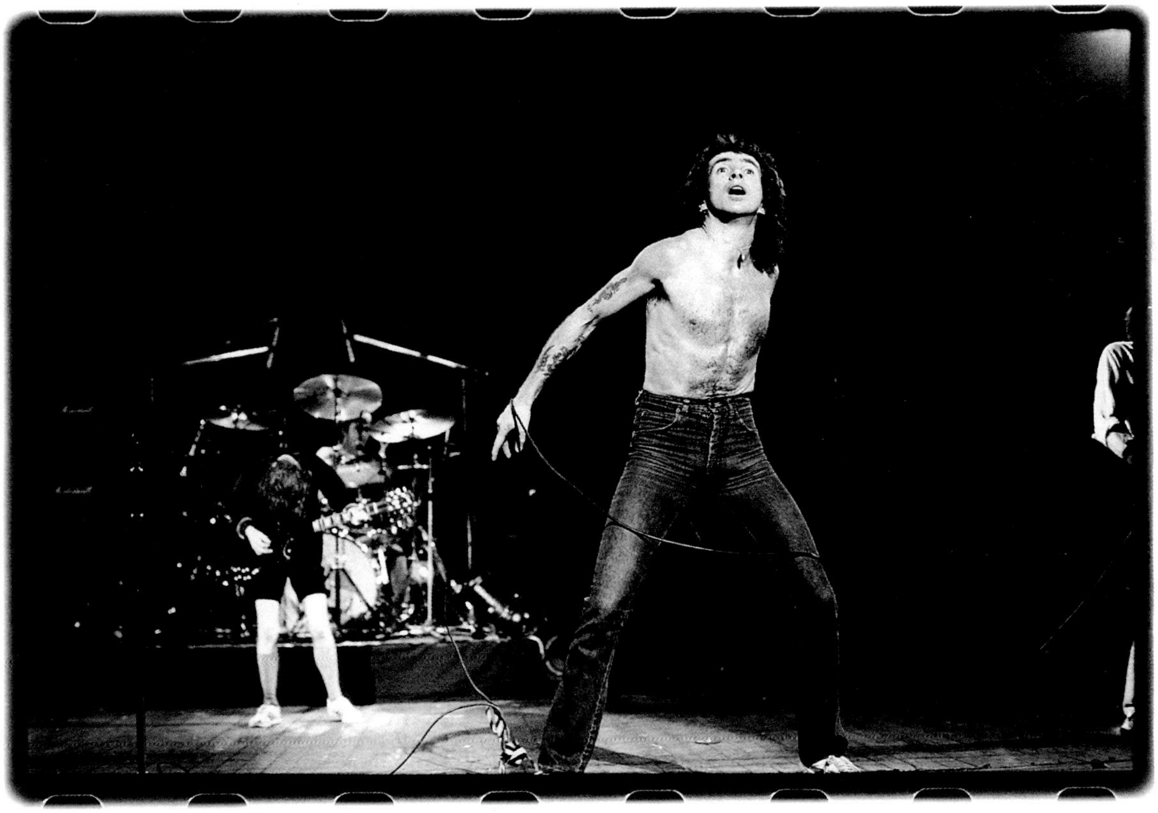

Bon Scott
Hammersmith Odeon, '79
The Power Age Tour

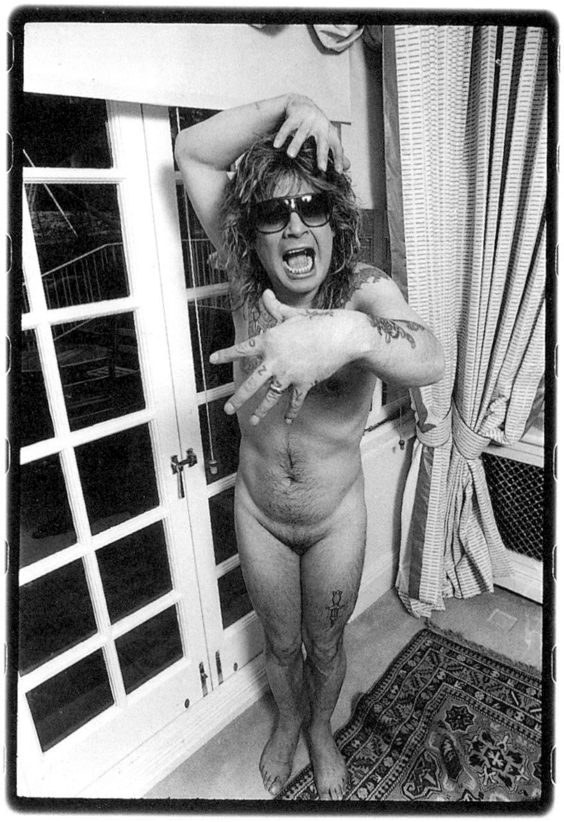

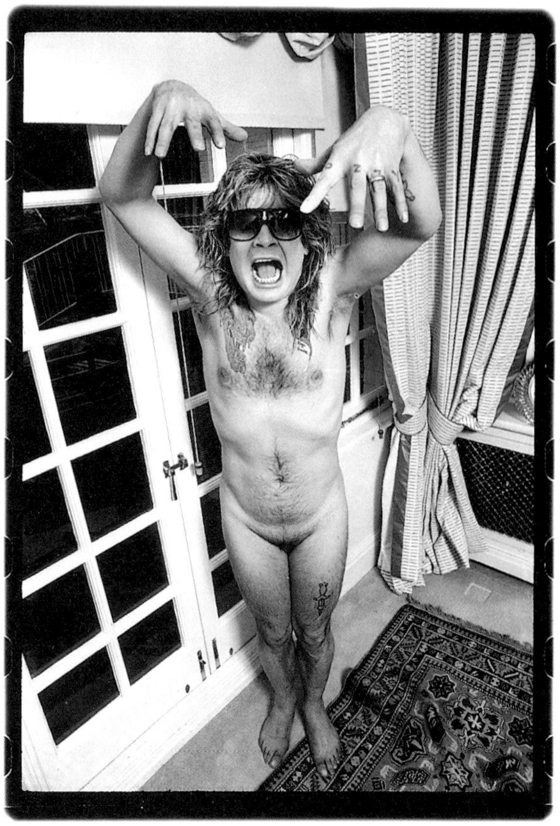

OZZY OSBOURNE

I had been hired - in July 1985 - to write Ozzy's official biography, *Diary of a Madman*, and had for several weeks been trying to get an interview together. But every time we scheduled a meeting something always seemed to scupper the plan at the last minute. . .First Ozzy was out of town; then he was in town but constantly "busy". One time, I turned up at his office and he had plainly forgotten all about the meeting and didn't show up. Another time, I turned up at the house he and his wife and manager, Sharon Osbourne, were renting in Berkeley Square, London, only to find both he and Sharon in bed together with the flu. I sat on the end of the bed and we chatted but we still didn't get our interview done.

Finally and much to my surprise, Ozzy offered to cook me Sunday lunch at his house, after which he promised we would get down to business and attempt to put his recollections down on tape.

The thought of Ozzy actually standing in the kitchen with his sleeves rolled-up and cooking me Sunday lunch was not half as surreal as the reality though.

I arrived in Berkeley Square at just after 1.00 p.m. the following Sunday and sure enough there he was, peeling potatoes and worrying about the roast in the oven, shelling peas and slicing carrots. "Can I help?" I asked. "No, no," he shook his head, "All under control. We're having traditional English Sunday roast - alright with you?"

"Definitely." I grabbed a seat at the table and waited to see what would happen next. Sharon and the nanny were busying themselves with the children - Aimee and Kelly - putting their coats on. They were going out to play in Hyde Park for an hour or so while Daddy finished cooking them lunch.

As the front door closed behind Sharon and the kids, Ozzy froze in his tracks. Literally, turned into a statue. I thought he was having a seizure or something.

"Everything alright, Ozzy?" I enquired.

"Sshh . . ."

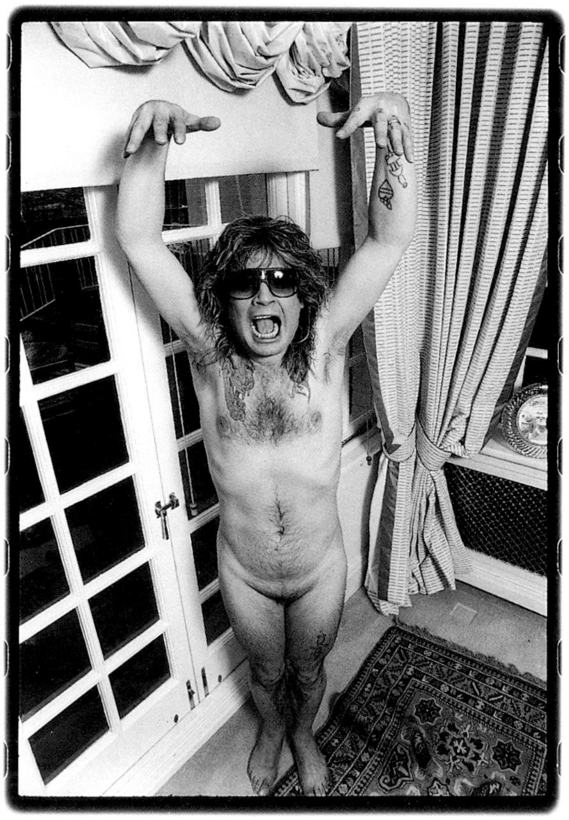

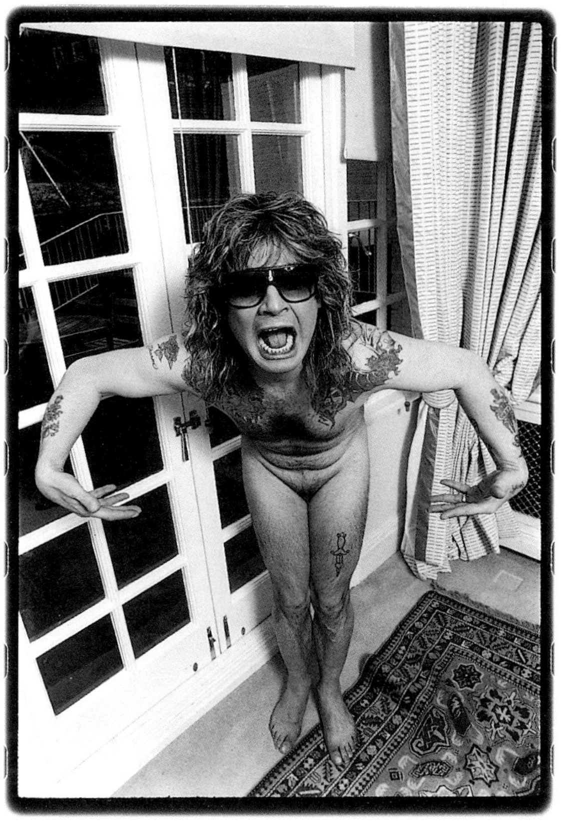

OZZY DRUNK, 11 A.M., HAMPSTEAD

We both lapsed into silence as outside we could hear car-doors slamming and the sound of ignitions being turned over. We listened in absolute silence as the car drove off. Ozzy still not moving a muscle, his whole being tuned to the sounds of Sharon's retreat.

He exhaled hugely. "Thank fuck for that" he sighed. "Do you wanna drink?"

I didn't know what to say. Before I could think of anything, he shoved a pint-glass in my hand, two-thirds full of white wine. 'Cheers!' he said, downing his own pint-glass of wine in one long, ungraceful haul, the wine spilling down his chin.

"Fucking hell, I needed that!" he cried as he set down his glass. "D'ya fancy another?" I had hardly started my own pint of wine. Ozzy had yanked another bottle from the refrigerator, and poured most of the contents into his glass. Down in one again. I began to worry about lunch.

. . .The lunch itself was a memorable affair. Ozzy had laden the table with roast beef, Yorkshire pudding, gravy, cabbage, carrots, peas and sprouts, and a large bowl of mash-potato lidded with melted cheese and garnished with parsley and thin slices of tomato. We filled our plates – Sharon, the nanny, and myself. Sharon filled Ozzy's plate for him as he didn't look like he was going to manage it. I didn't know how many pint-glasses of wine he put down by the time Sharon came home.

Five minutes into the meal, Ozzy's head very gently lowered itself into his plate until it came to rest in the mash potatoes. Ozzy began to snore, the gravy bubbling around his nose.

"Is he alright?" I asked no one in particular for what must have been the 10th time that day. "Oh yeah, just leave him," said Sharon. We sat there and ate the entire lunch while Ozzy lay with his head in his plate, snoring.

MICK WALL

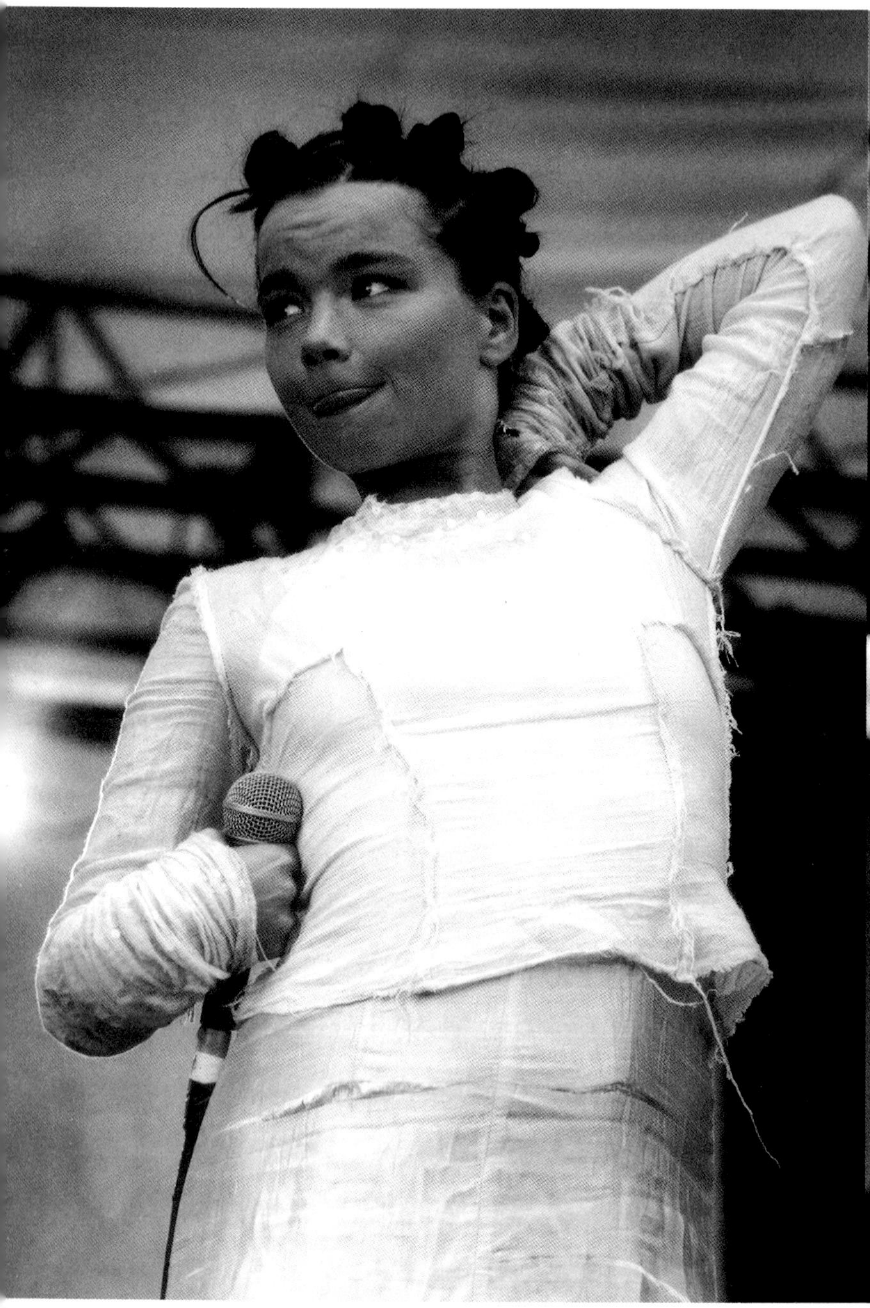
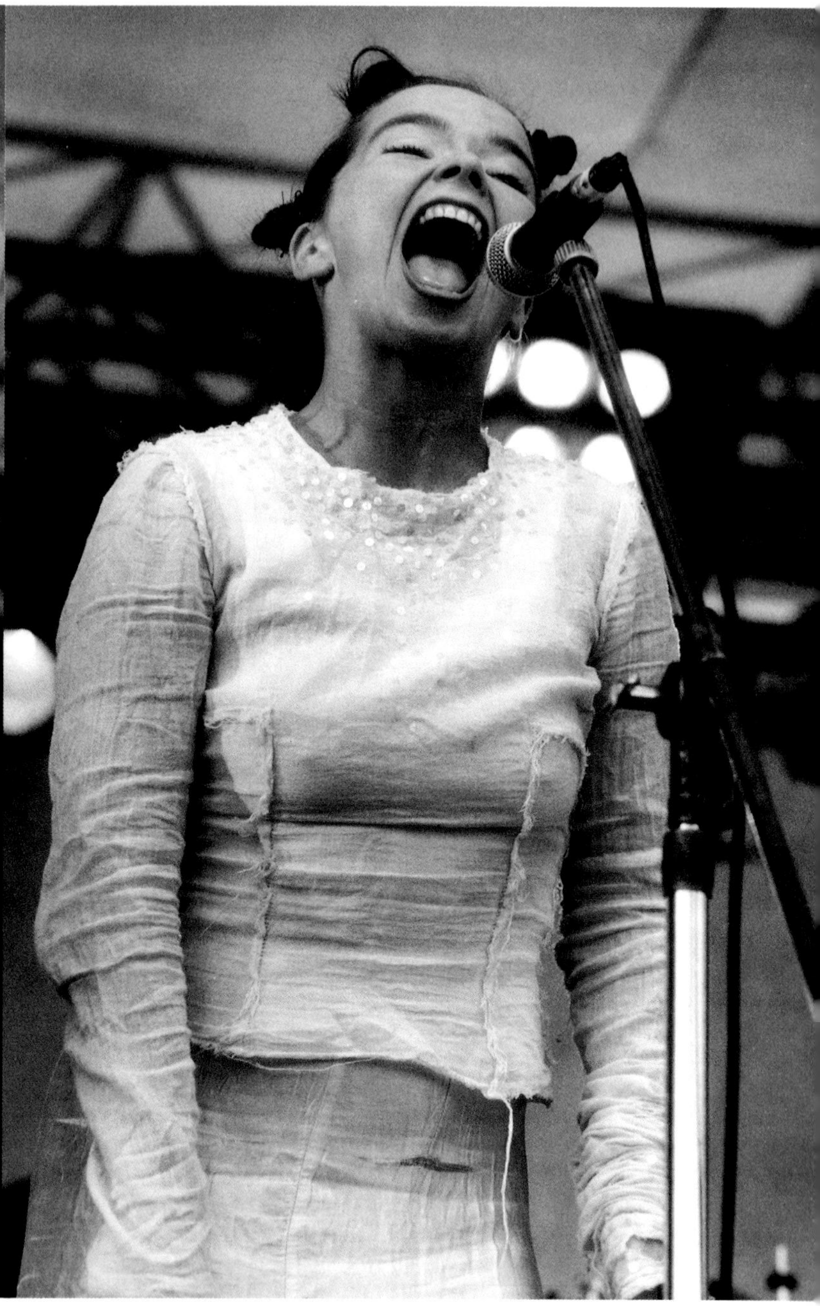

BJÖRK

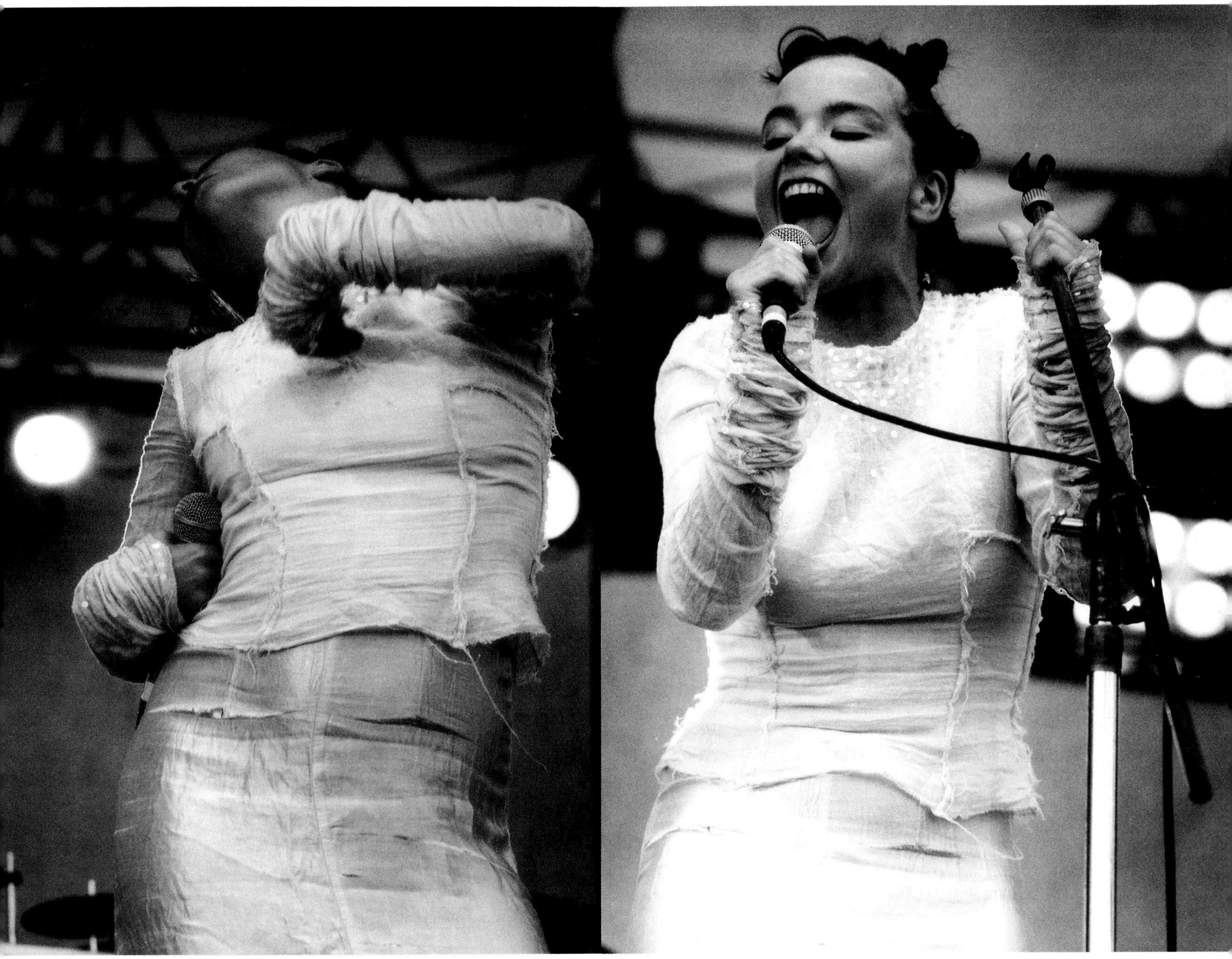

BJÖRK, MELBOURNE, '94

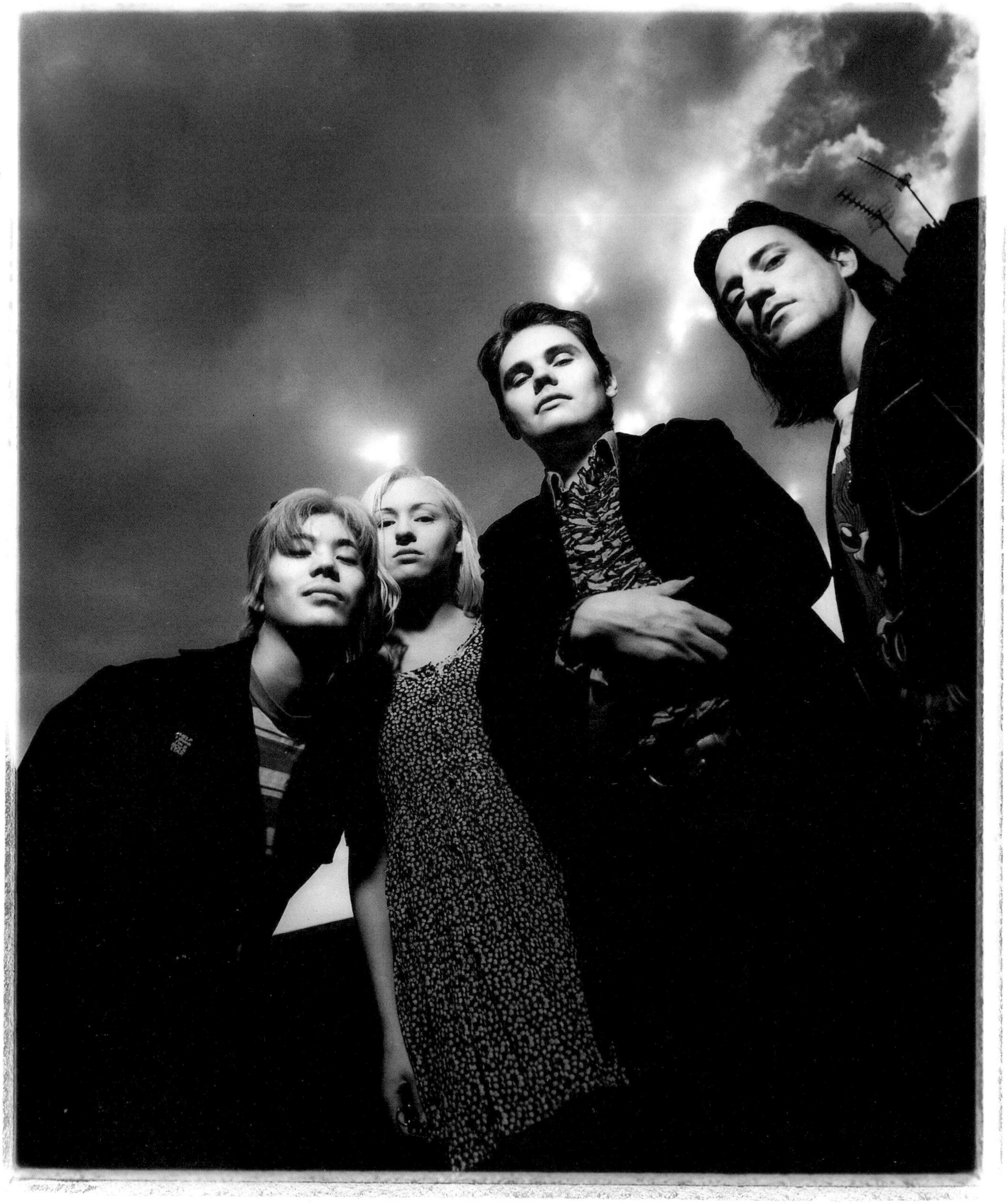

Smashing Pumpkins
London

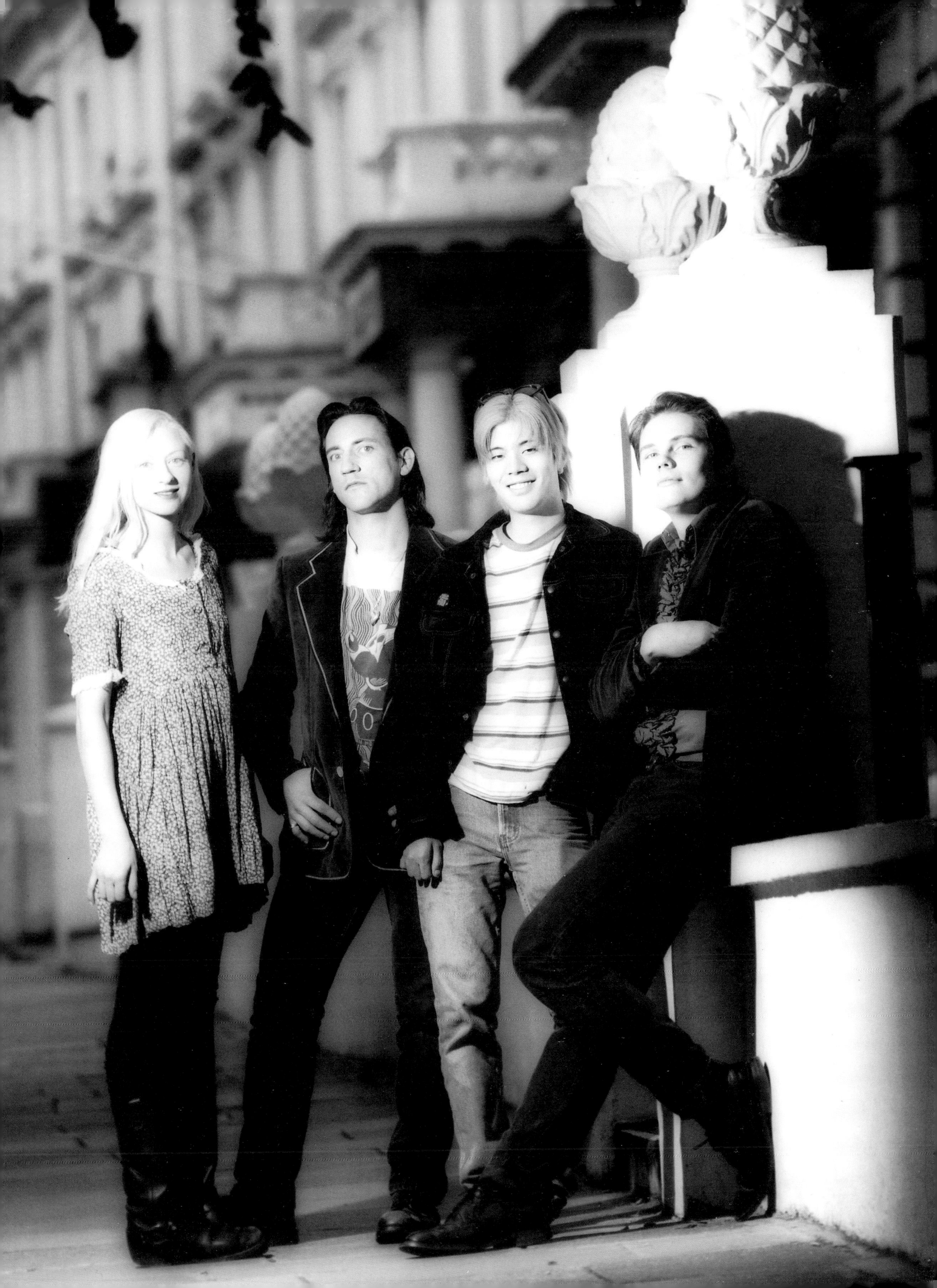

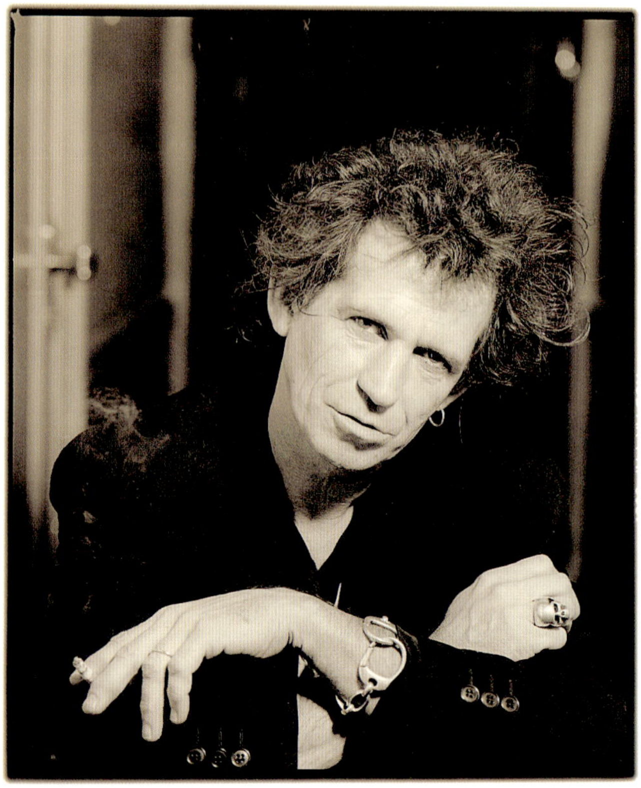

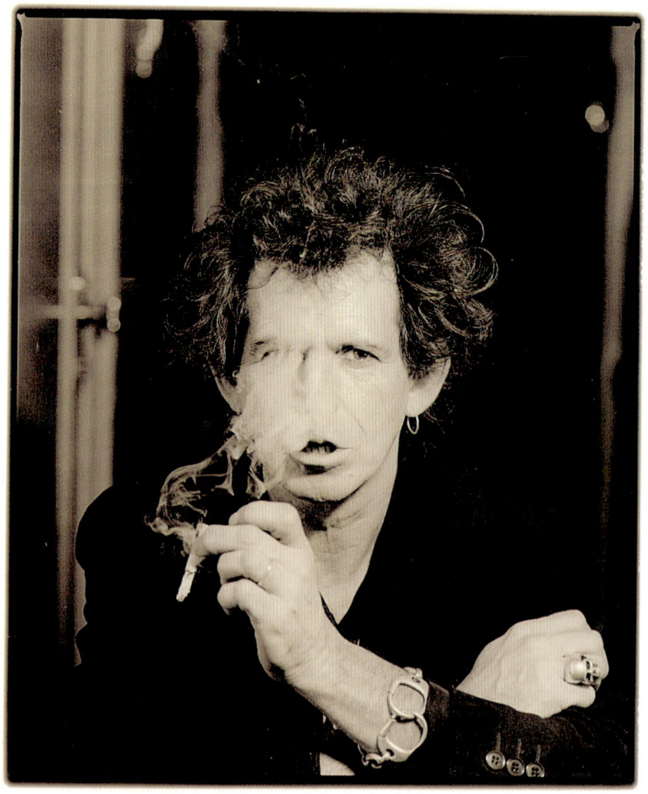

Keith Richards
Denmark

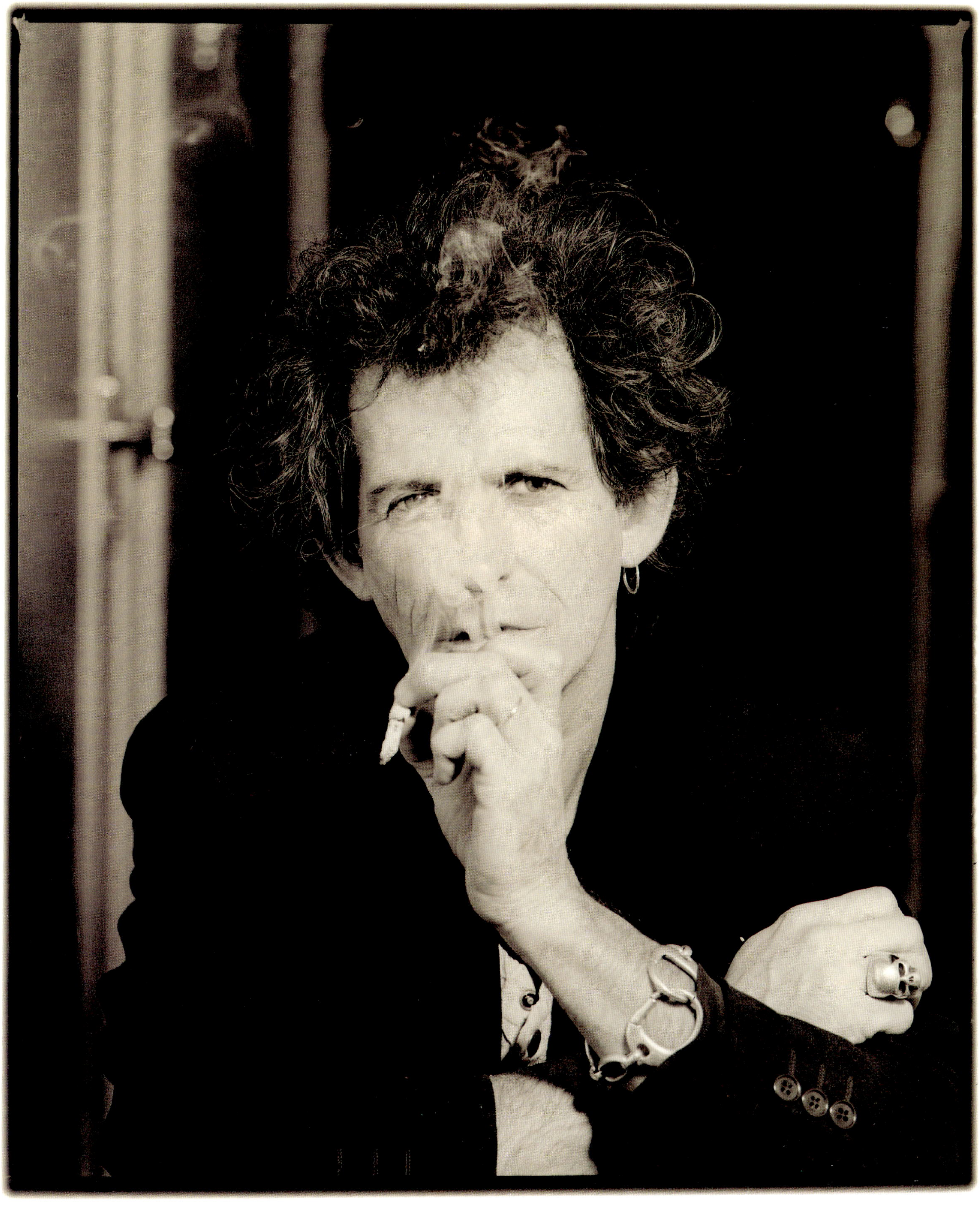

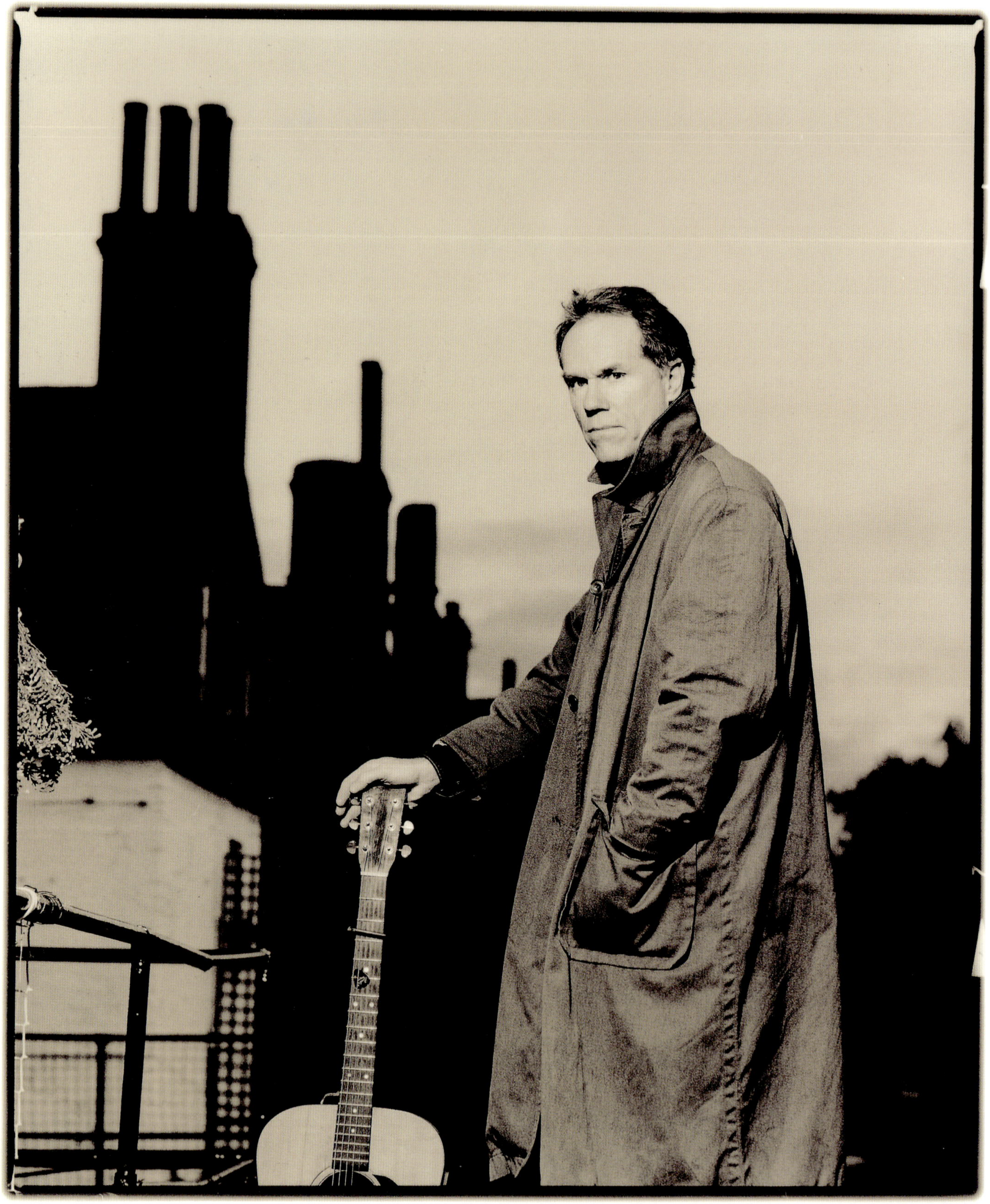

Loudon Wainwright III
London, October '95

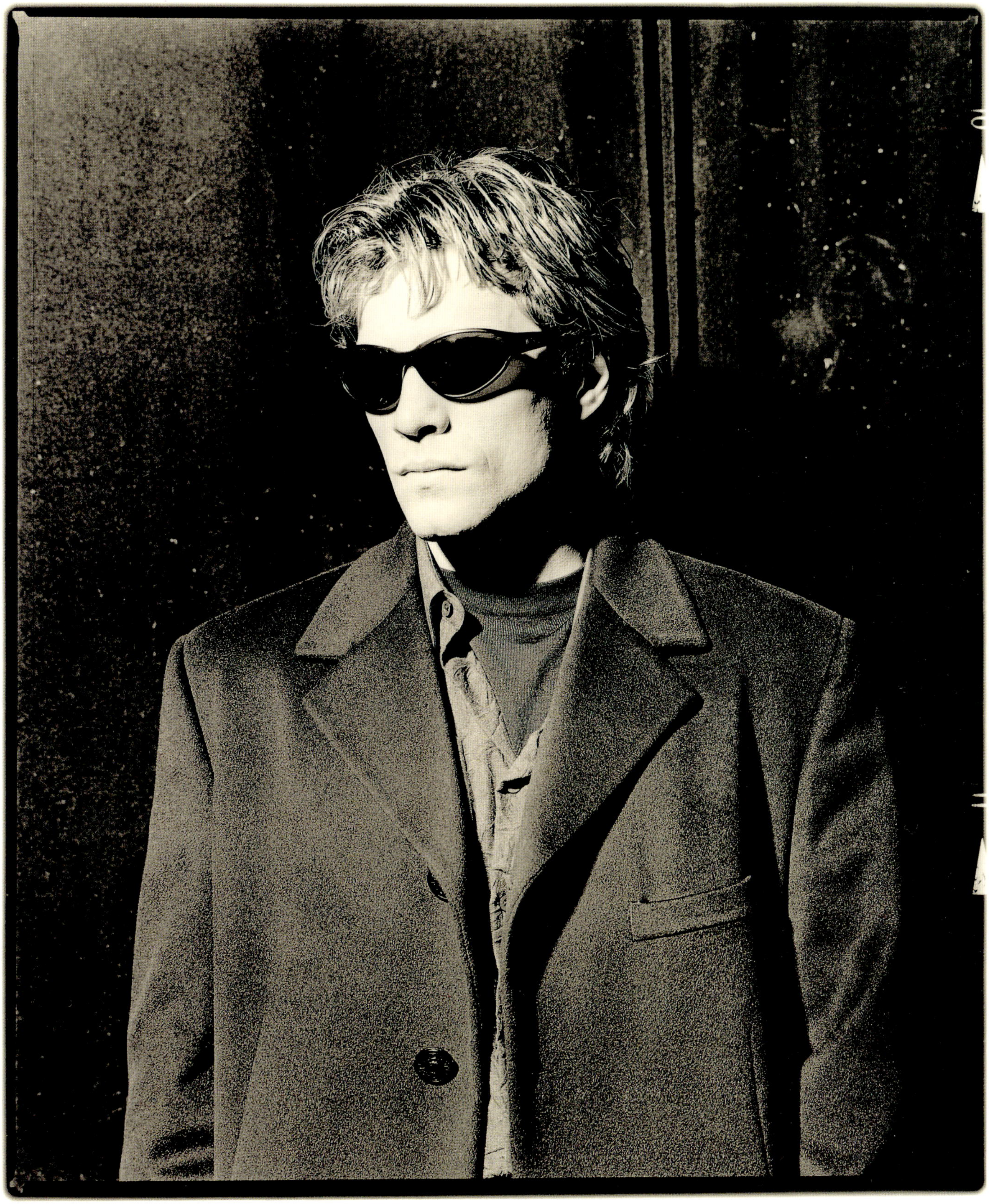

Jon Bon Jovi
London, '96

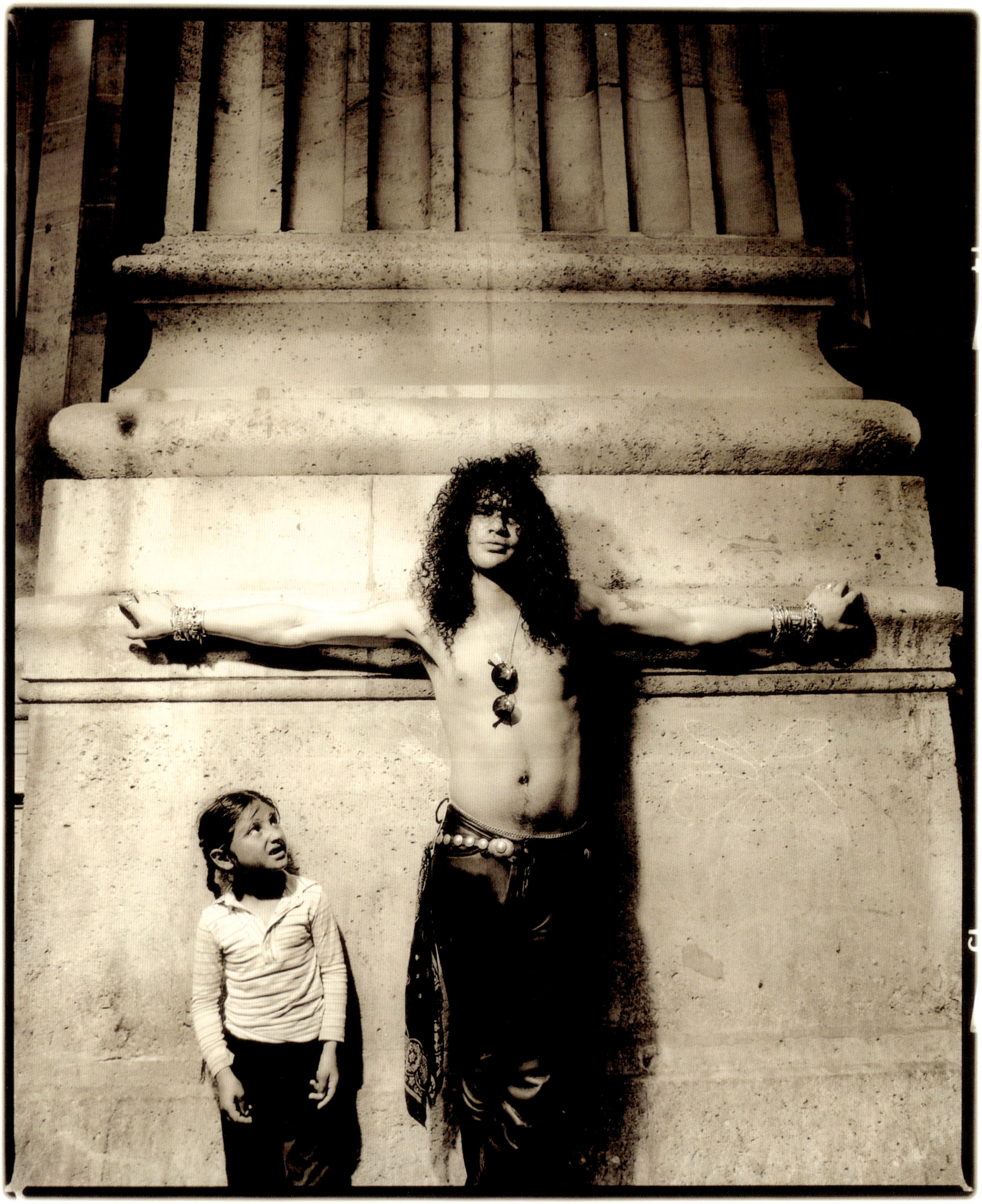

Slash
Du Nord Station
Paris, July '95

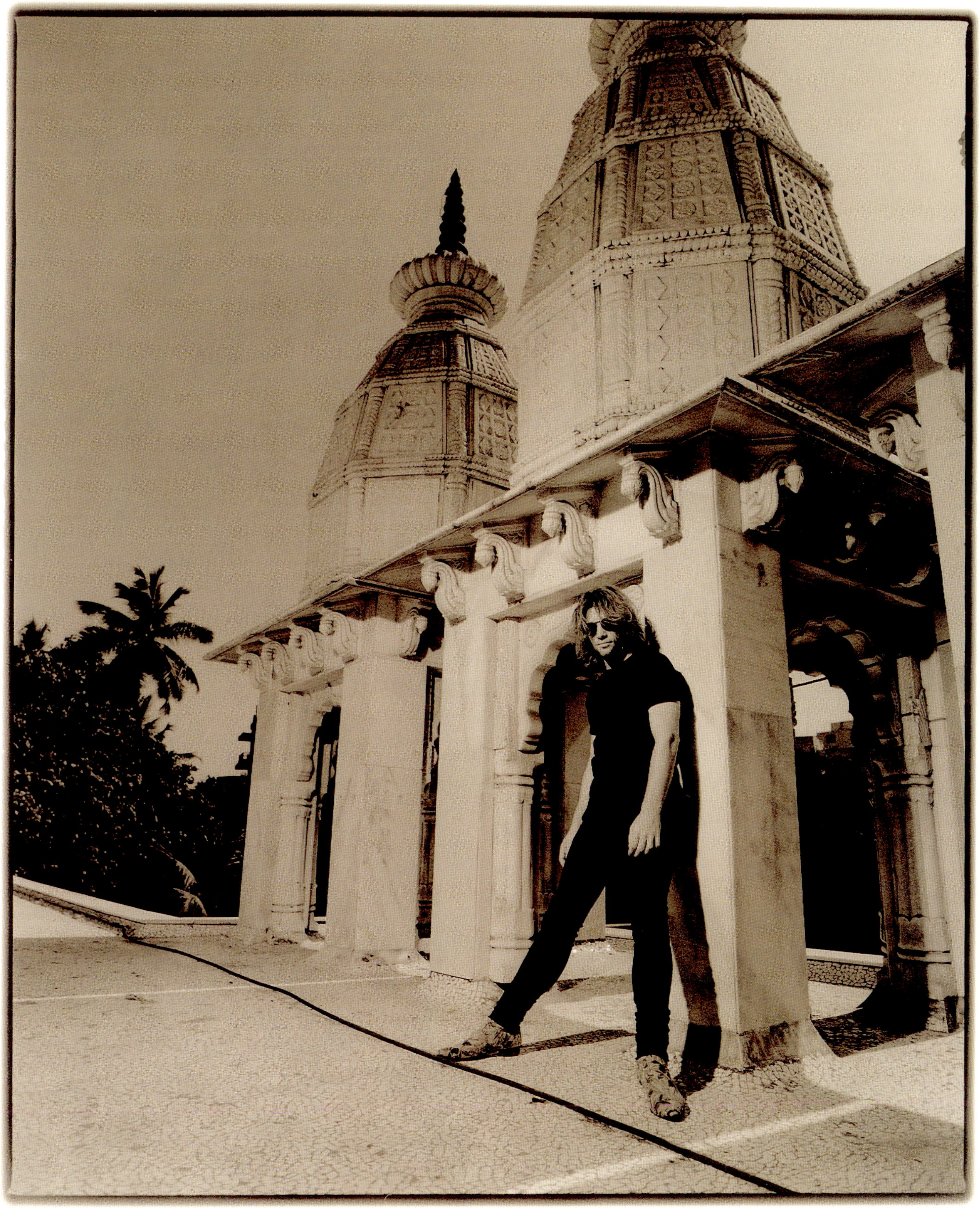

Jon Bon Jovi
Hari Krishna Temple
Juhu, Bombay, '95

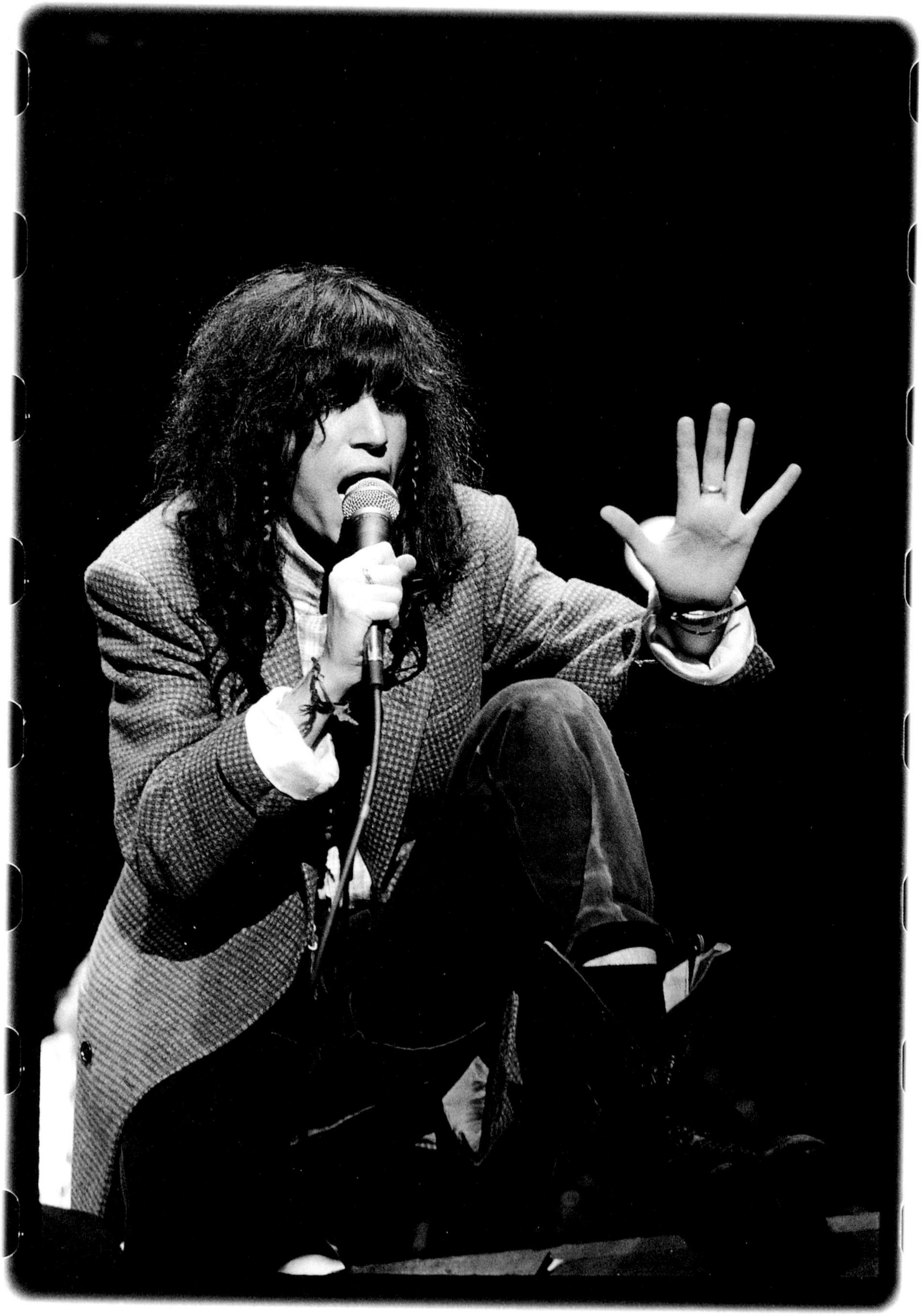

Patti Smith
Reading Festival

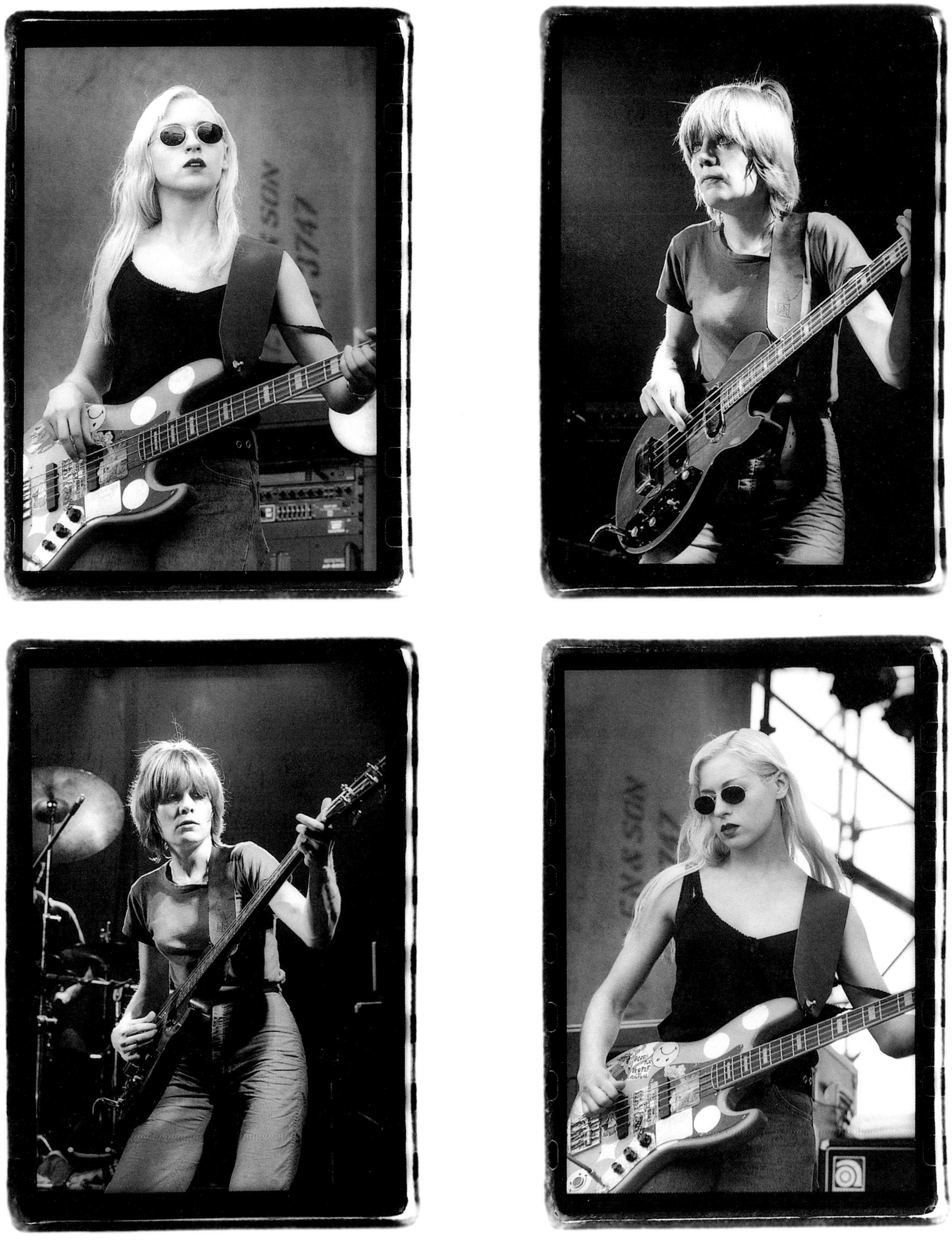

D'arcy Of Smashing Pumpkins
And Tina Weymouth

george harrison

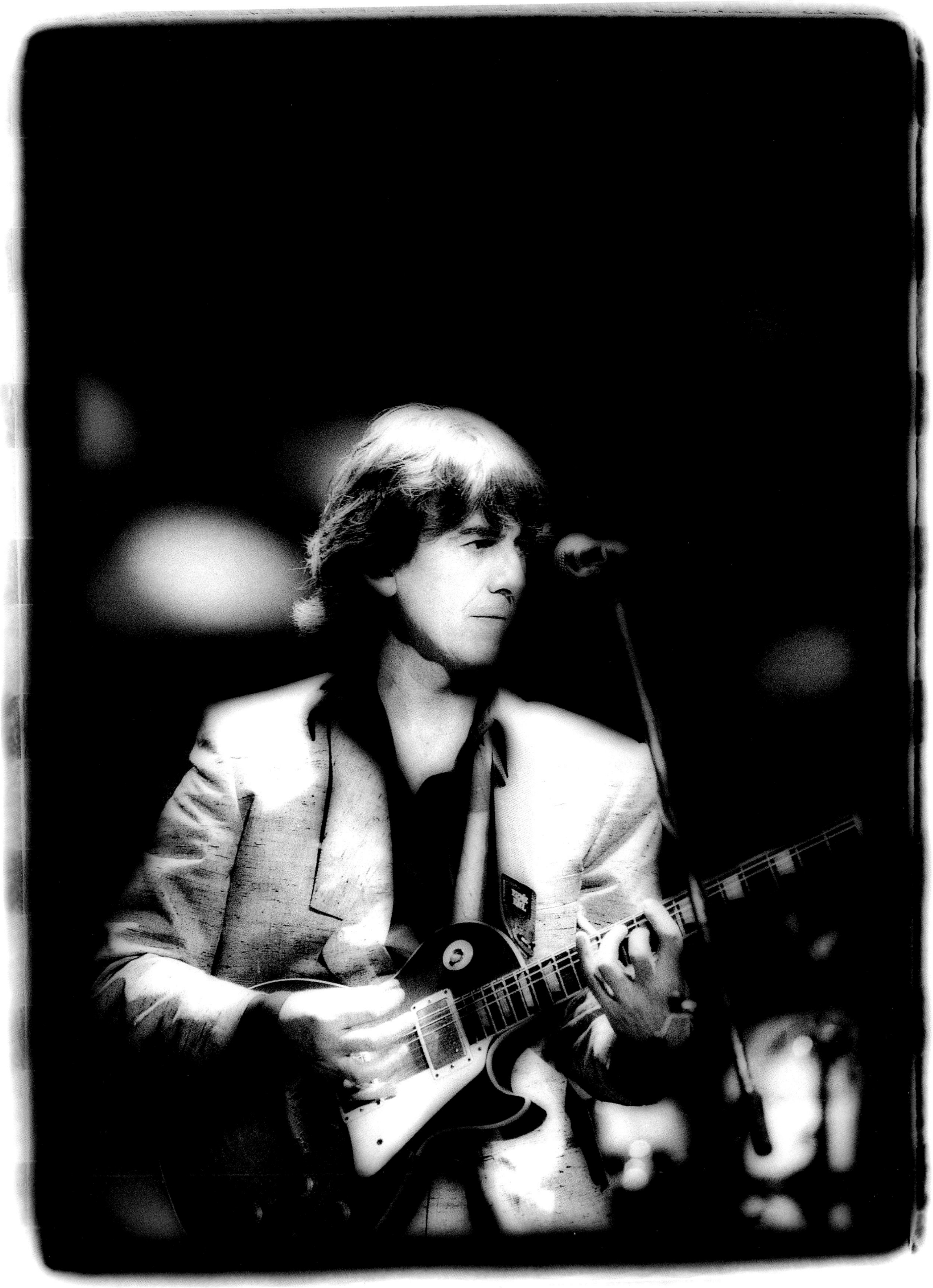

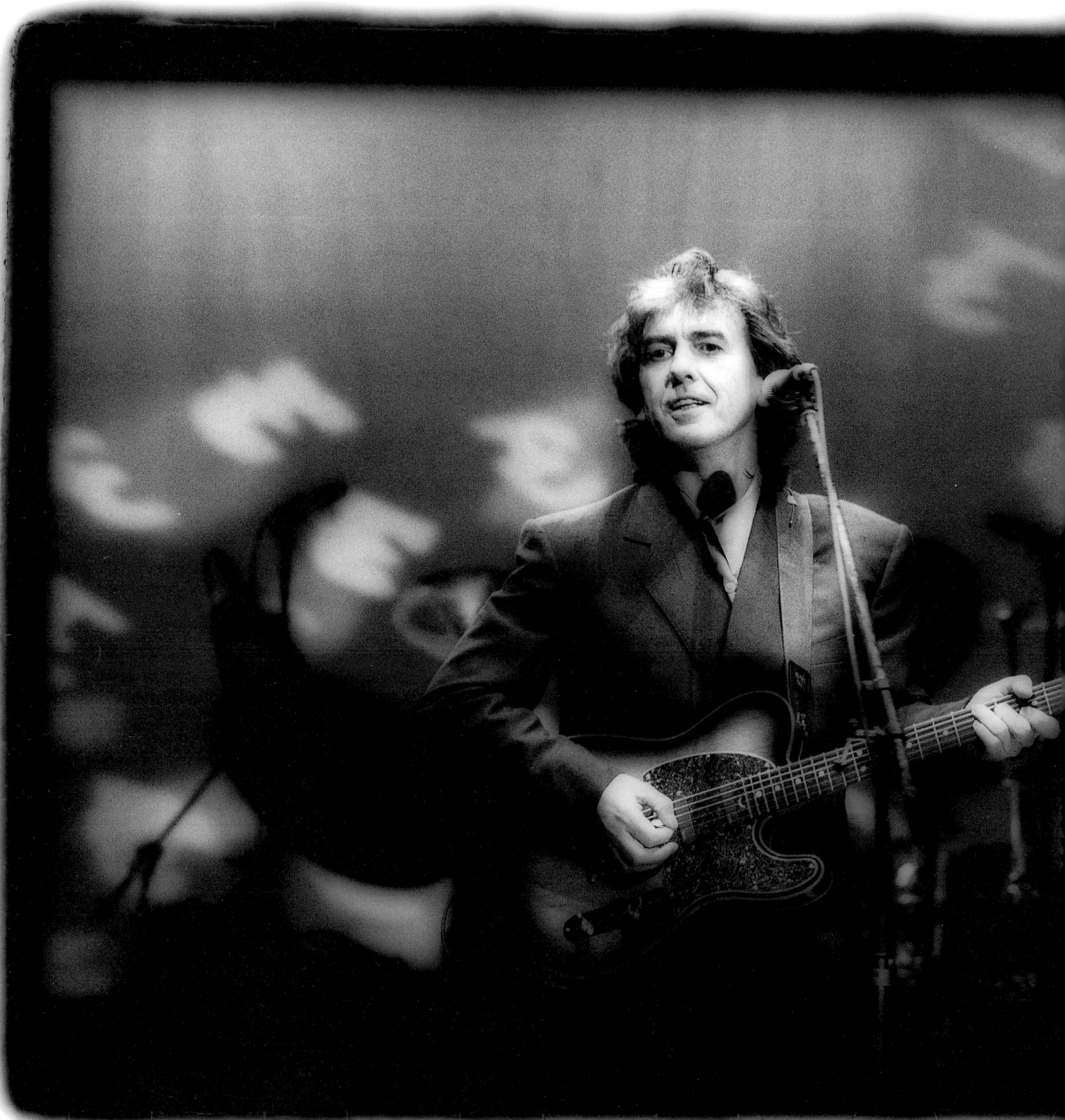

George Harrison, Osaka Castle, December '91

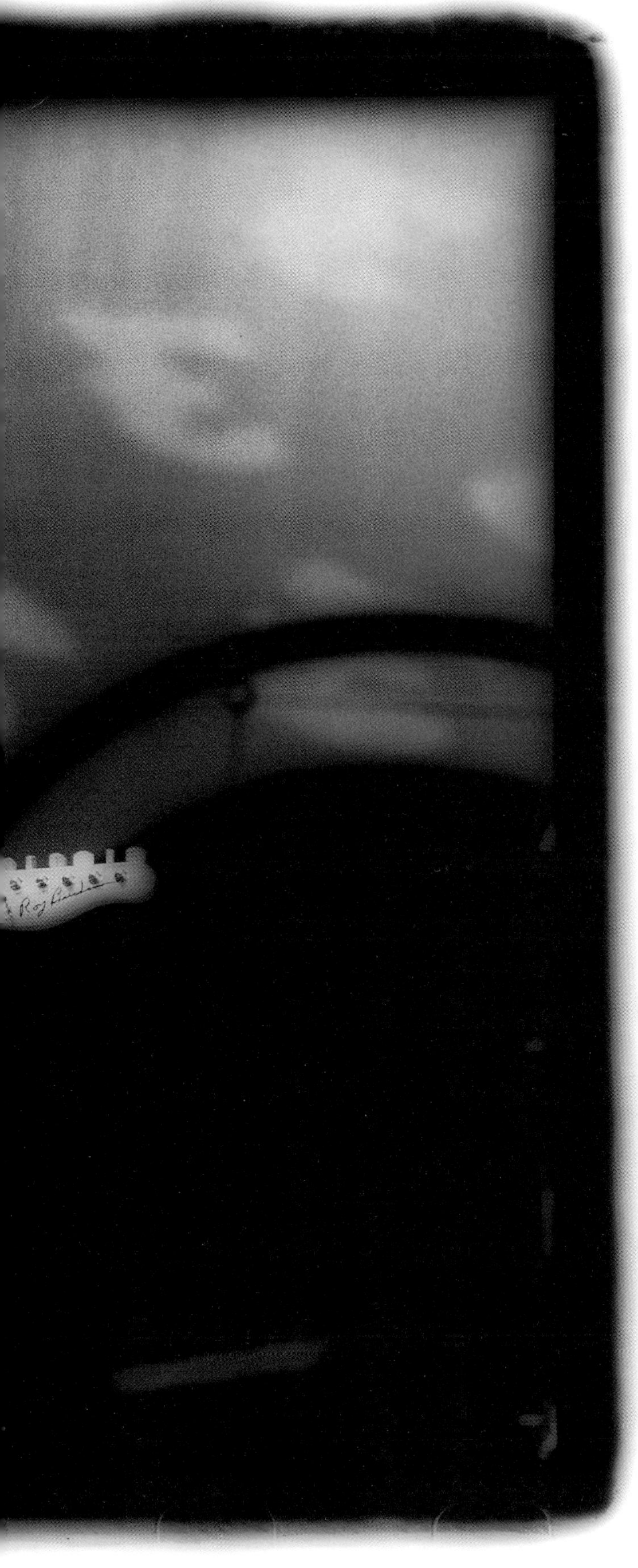

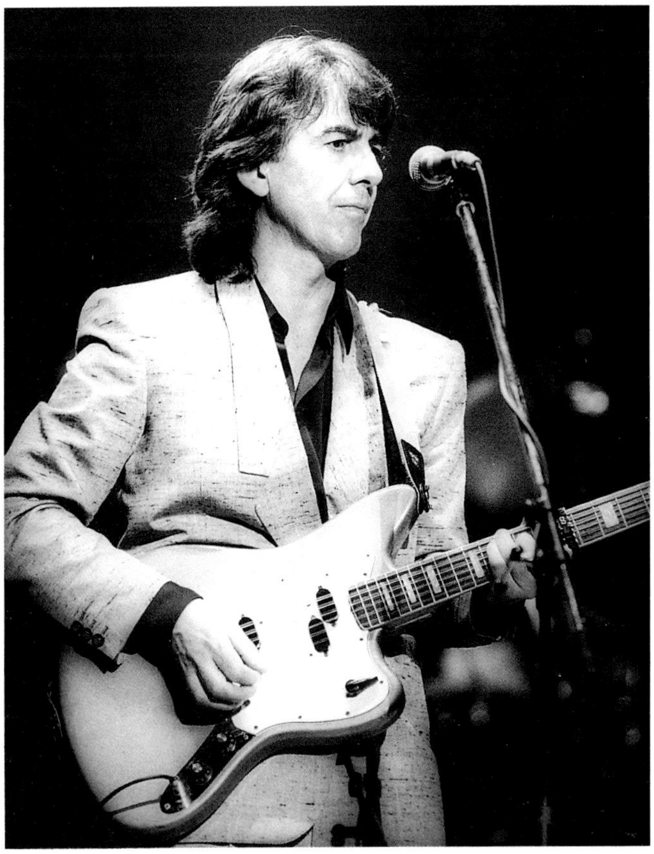

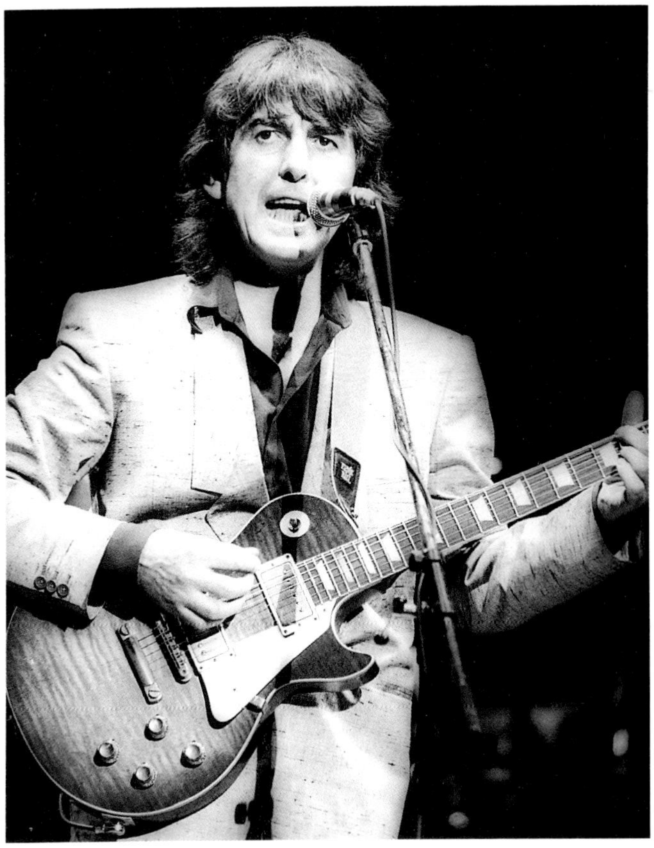

steve clark
def leppard

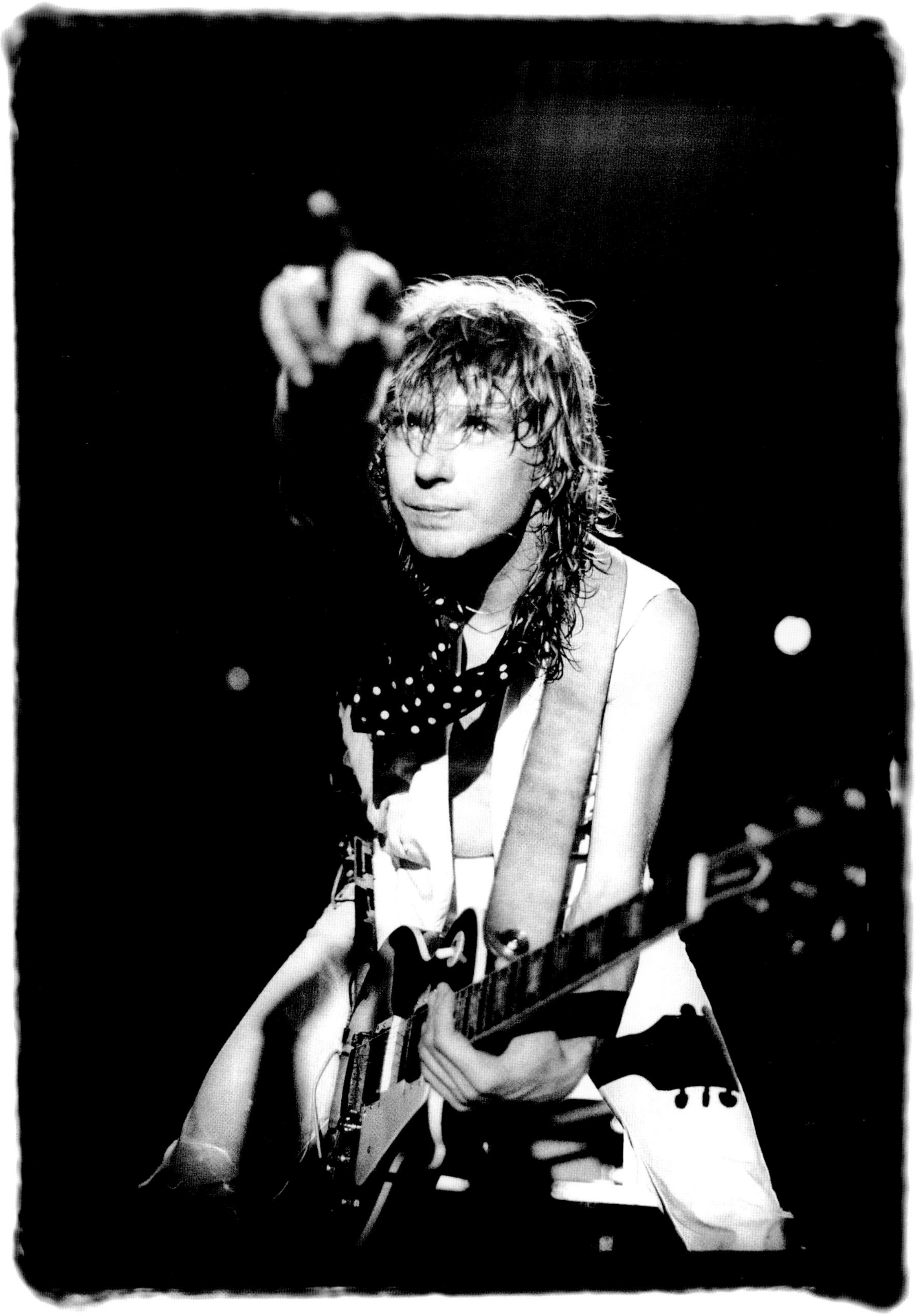

Steve Clark
New York, '83

STEVE CLARK
Memories of a Stray...

2:00 a.m... Boston or maybe Denver... a ring on the phone. I pick it up.

"What are you doing?" Steve asks.

"Nothing, the hotel bar is closed," I reply.

"Listen, I've got some vodka and stuff... can I come up?" Of course, he can come up, but before I can say so he's already backpedaling, apologizing before he's even done anything. "I mean, not if you're doing anything... if you're not up for it, it's alright, you know... not if you're not, you know..."

A lot of the way Steve used to speak, the things he tried to say, would come out backwards, like someone trying to leave the room without taking their eyes off you.

He was always nervous. I never met a less prepossessing rock star.

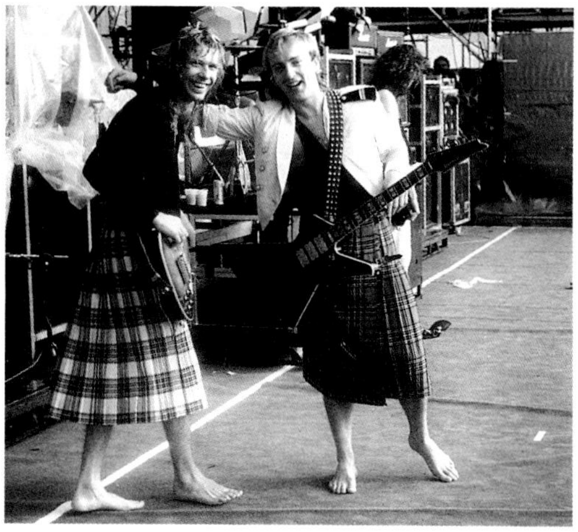

What was unusual about Steve Clark was that here was someone who, on the surface at least, appeared to have no problems at all accepting his status as a millionaire rock star - that's what a band like Def Leppard was built for, wasn't it? But underneath the brash, blond-streaked exterior was a deeply confused and unhappy figure. Success, to Steve, seemed less a reward and more of a burden, a constant reminder not of his talents but of his limitations.

At the time, I was truly baffled. What was wrong with this guy? Here was an enigma worth unraveling, I thought.

So... we had become close. Not gradually, but all at once. Like you do. Drunk close. We had something in common: booze and drugs. And anything else that would keep your mind off the inevitable sigh of tomorrow. . .

Years later, it's hard for me to remember why I was like that, let alone why Steve Clark was the way he was. These days, they would call it "denial". I had my own cable TV show, was the author of many well-thumbed articles and books etc. and always wore my contact lenses and made sure I didn't put on too much weight. What I really liked to do though was get fucked up.

And Steve was who he was - the fading star in a band already reliant on the other guitarist in the line-up, Phil Collen, a fabulously gifted technician whose virtues (a strictly teetotaler, non-smoking pagan with a passion for physical exercise) only served to point up Steve's weaknesses. At least, in Steve's eyes.

But to get back to the story.

By the latter stages of Def Leppard's 1988 *Hysteria* world tour, it was not unusual for Steve and I to end the evening in one or the other's room, putting away the vodka and cranberry juice while we snorted coke and smoked endless cigarettes, telling each other ludicrous stories of rock and woe that in most cases we had already told each other many, many times already, like you do, until it was time to pretend to go to bed...

"Don't tell the others," he would repeat like a mantra as he chopped us out another couple of fat ones on the coffee table.

The end of this particular night was no different – made memorable, though, for two things. The first was Steve's offer to loan me some money. At the time, I was going through a brief period of financial security and was certainly not in need of a loan of any kind. Nor had I suggested otherwise to Steve. But somehow, the offer was made.

"You know, if you ever need some dough, you know you can come to me," he had said. I'll never forget his face. Sincere as a new-born foal, drunken and drooling as the village slosh pot, his heart-wings flapping in the smoke-fugged breeze.

"Thanks man, but I really don't need any money," I said. "I have my own money." Somewhere in my out-of-it-ness, I had felt somewhat slighted though. I did not want his money. I was not a groupie, etc. I conveyed some of this to him, by way of shrugs and grunts and much chugging on cigarettes.

He understood.

"No, I mean, I don't know... if you needed, like, fifty grand or something... you know... you only have to ask. That's all."

He poured more drinks. Fifty grand. I lit another cigarette. FIFTY GRAND. He wasn't kidding.

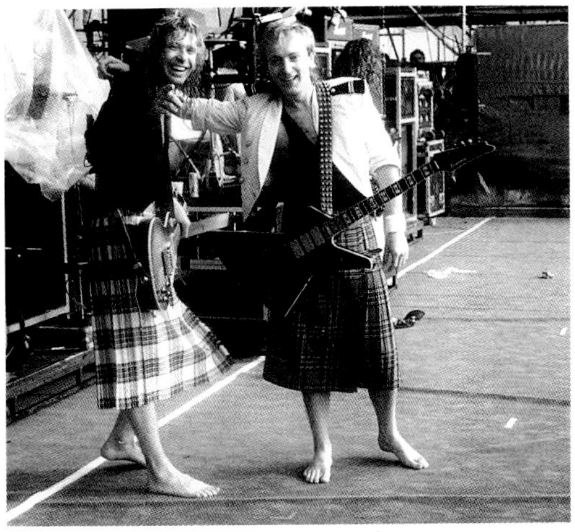

But neither was I. I stood up.

"IF YOU THINK I'M JUST SITTIN' HERE BECAUSE YOU'RE WHO YOU ARE THEN I DON'T FUCKING KNOW WHAT I'M FUCKING DOING HERE!" I yelled, drunk and stoned.

He looked at me. Tears welled in his eyes.

"No, no, no, no, no..." He stood up and put his arms around me; did his best to reassure me. No slight intended. All done with the best intentions. I acted hurt and pissed off. Then he went to take a piss and by the time he'd come back, we'd both forgotten about it and were onto the next thing, whatever that was...

The SECOND reason that particular evening was so memorable is because it was the first (and last) time I ever slept with a rock star. What happened was he was asleep on my bed. Out with drink still in hand. I tried to wake him but it was impossible.

I took his shoes off, loosened the collar of his shirt, undid his belt buckle, pushed him over onto his side and stuck a pillow under the side of his head, put a waste-paper basket over by his side of the bed, rolled the rest of the duvet around him, then lay down on the other side of the bed and turned out the overhead light.

Two seconds later, it was morning. Or what seemed like two seconds later. It might have been one and a half. I remember the bedside phone going – a wake-up call from the tour manager. The phone was on Steve's side of the bed. A hand snaked out and answered it.

"Uh... uhhh... uhhhh..."

The phone dropped from his hand and fell to the floor with a loud clatter. It made both of us sit up. He looked at me, puzzled.

"Mick," he said, "I know we're mates, but what the fuck are you doing in my bed?"

"Steve," I said, "it's not your bed. It's mine."

"Aarrrggggghhhhh!" he screamed, genuinely shocked it seemed. He dashed out of the bed, pulling up his jeans as he went, then banged out of the door. Two minutes later, there was a frantic knocking. I reluctantly got up and answered it. It was Steve.

"Are my fucking shoes in there?"

"Oh... yeah." I went to get them. I passed them to him.

He looked around the room. "This is your room? What happened? Did I pass out?"

"No, you fucked me. What do you think fucking happened?" I said.

"Alright, alright... BUT DON'T TELL THE BAND!!!"

I went back to bed.

Mick Wall

the black crowes

The Brothers Robinson
London
'92

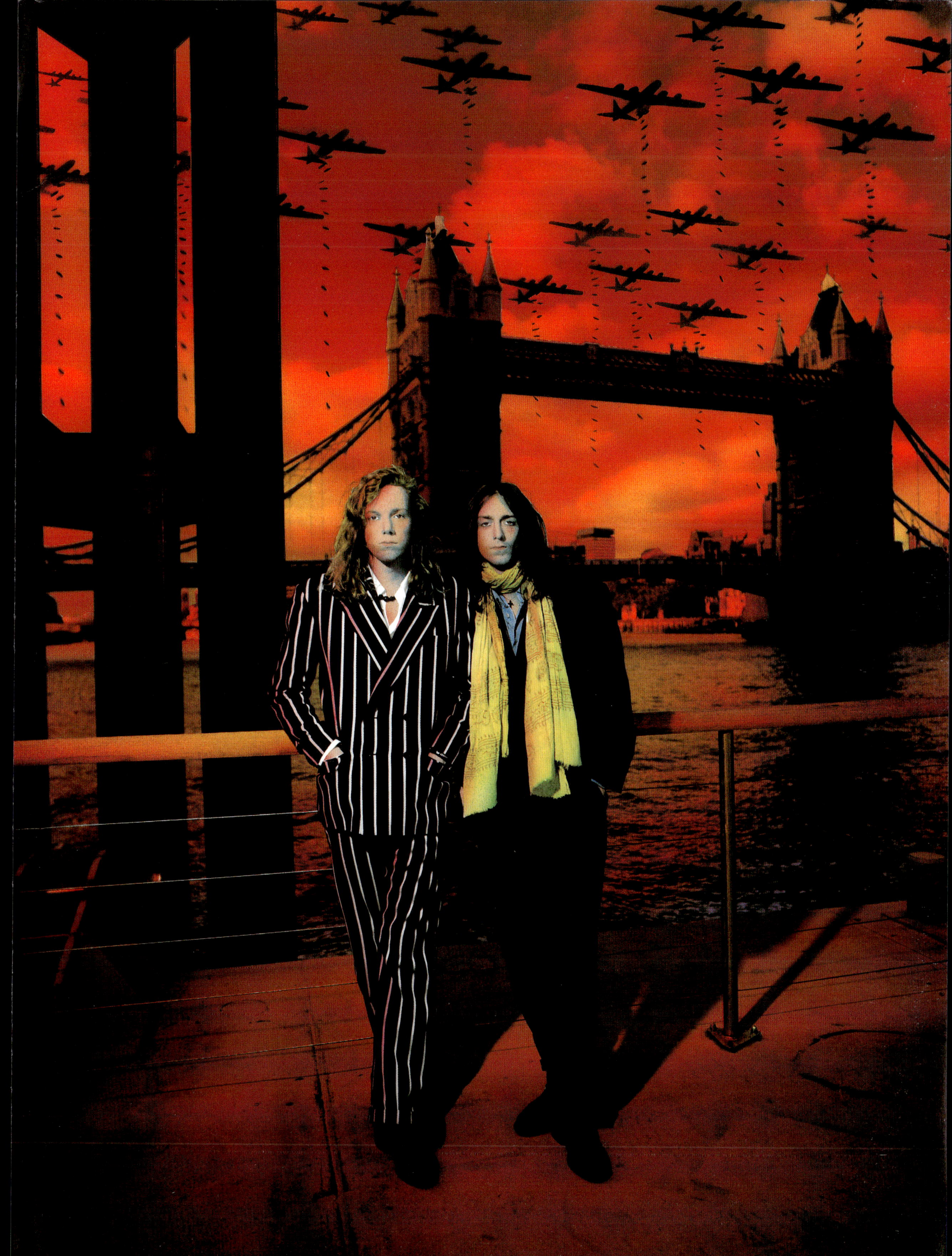

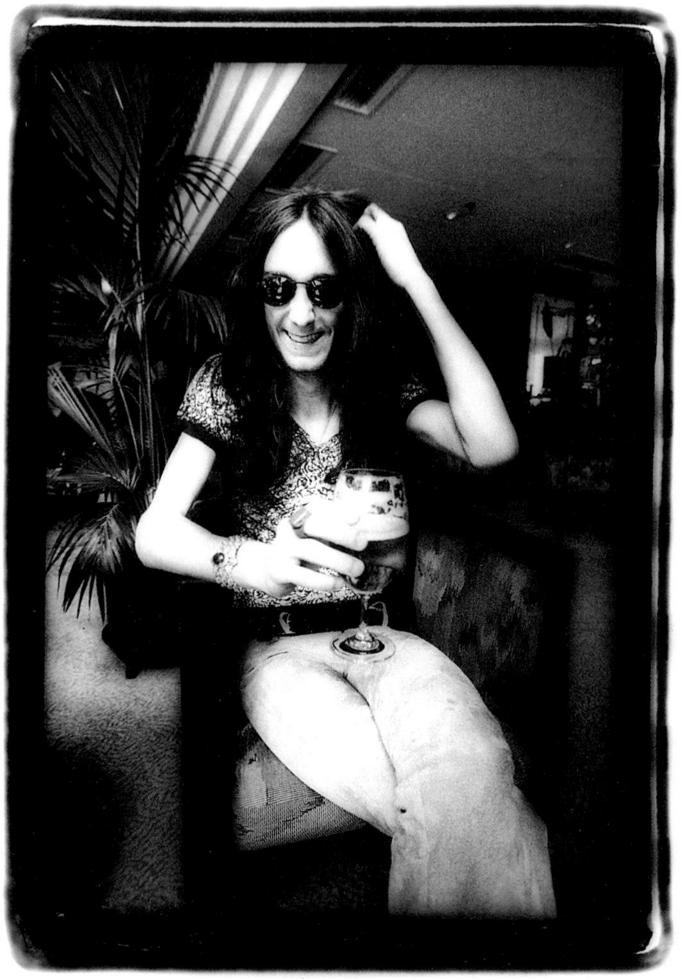

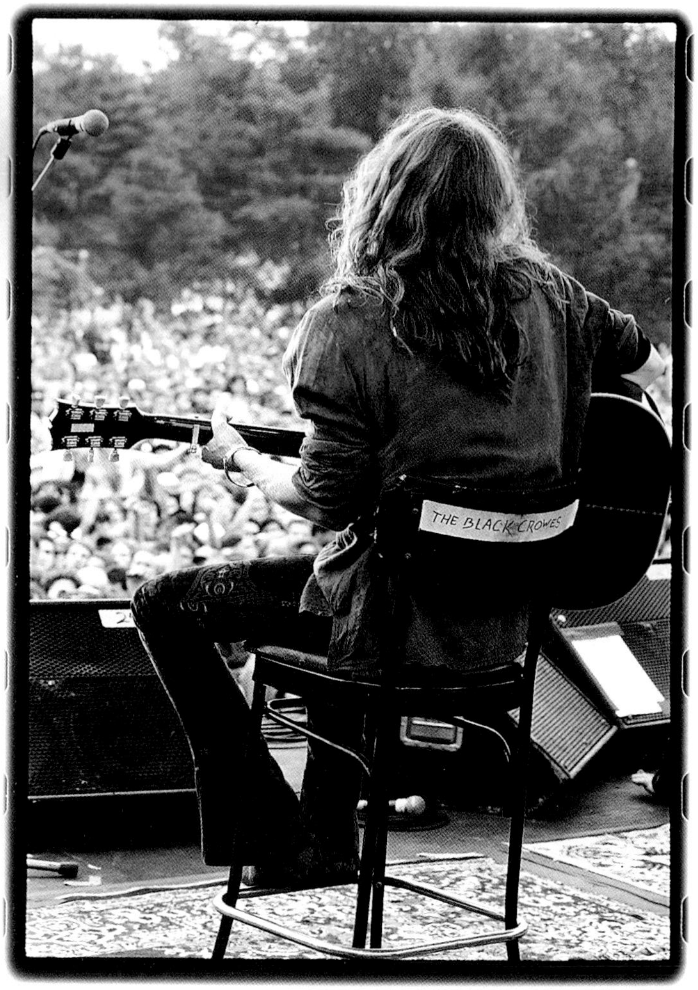

CHRIS ROBINSON, VIENNA, MAY '93

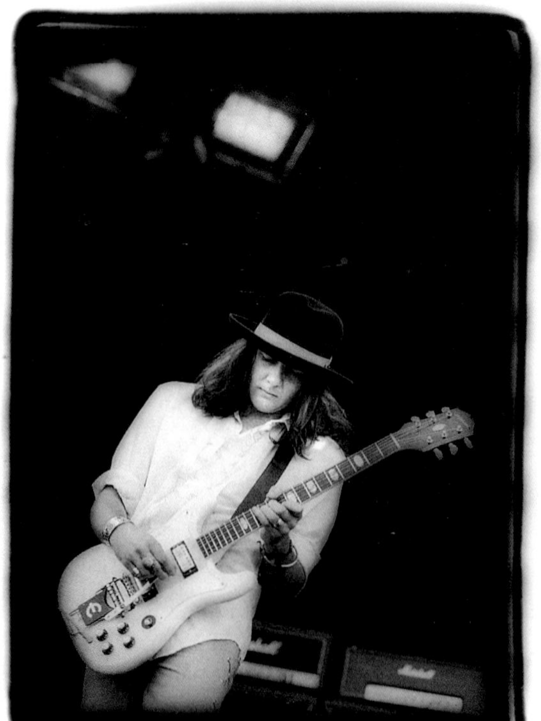

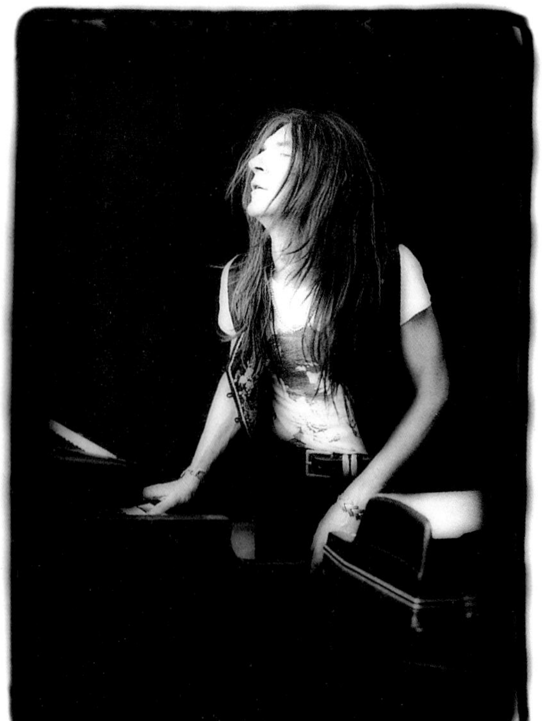

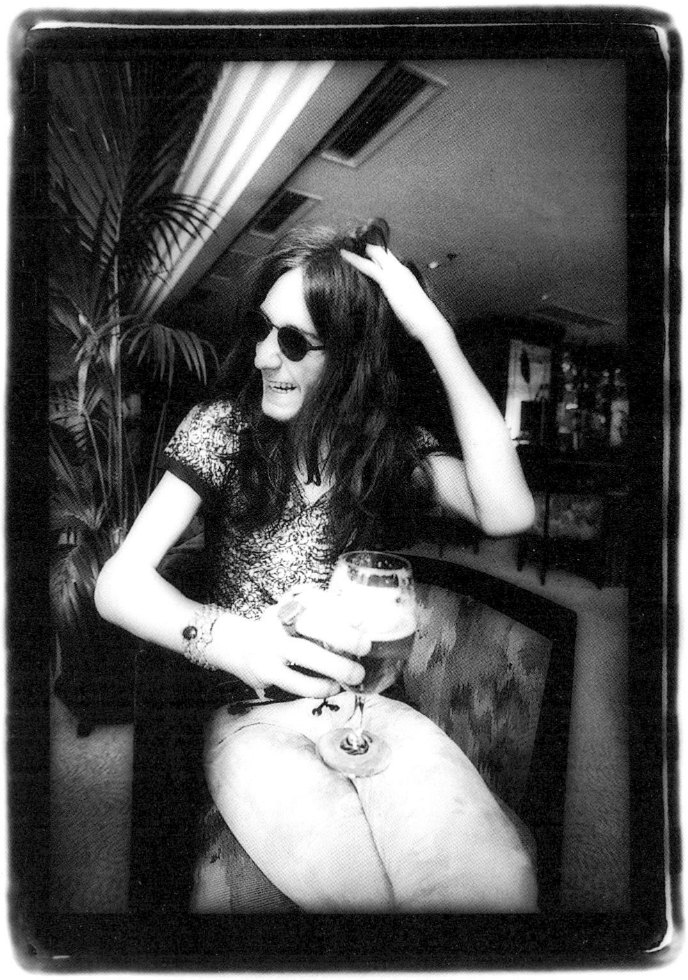

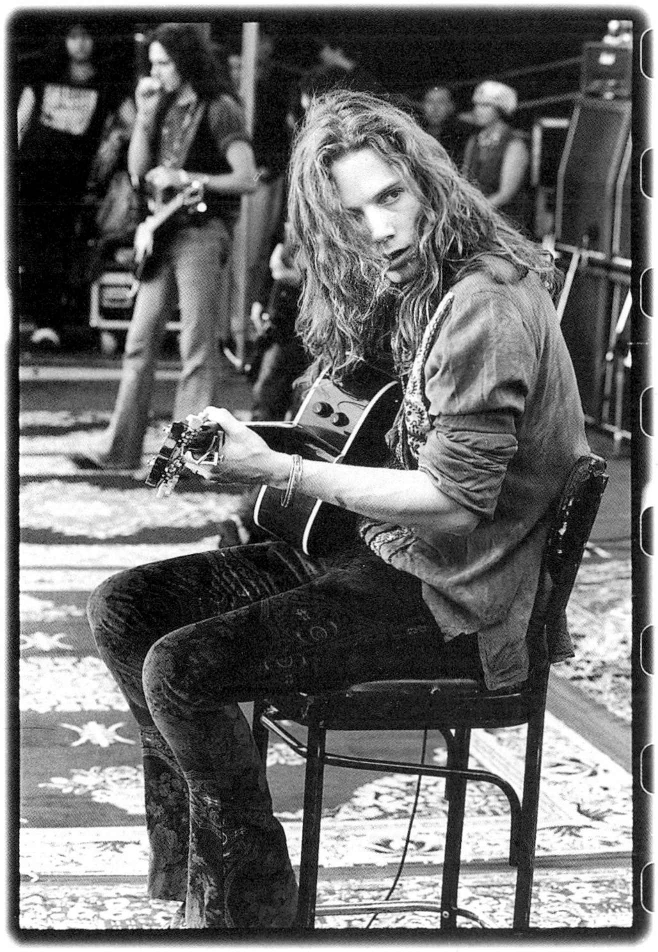

Rich Robinson, Toronto, '92

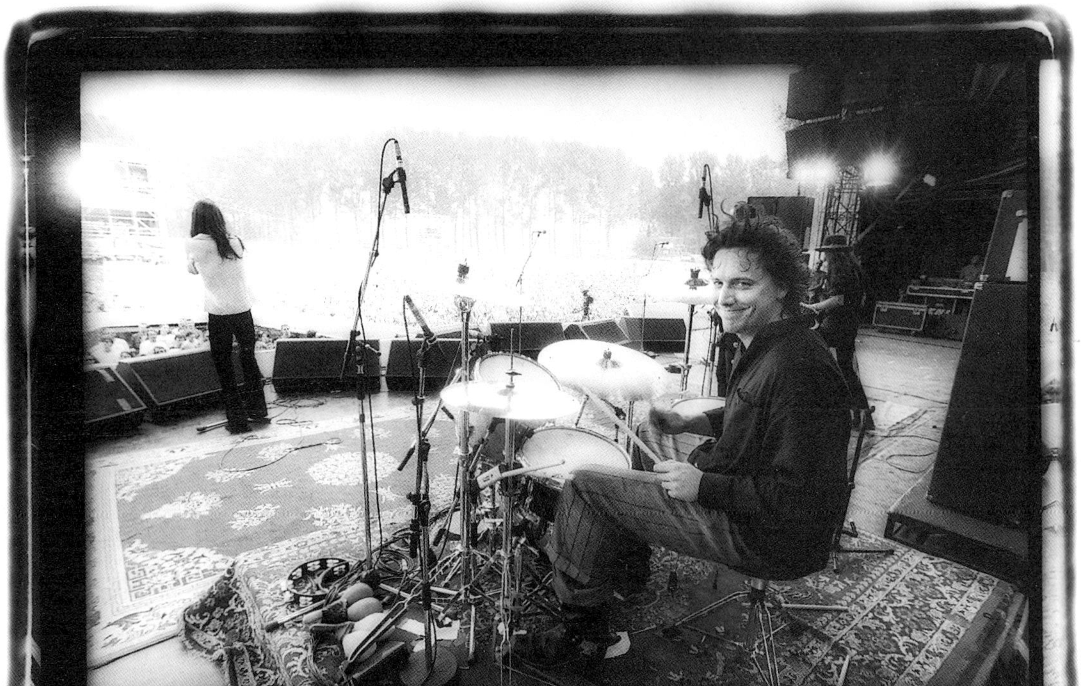

Right:
Steve Gorman

Left:
Marc Ford
Ed Hawrysch

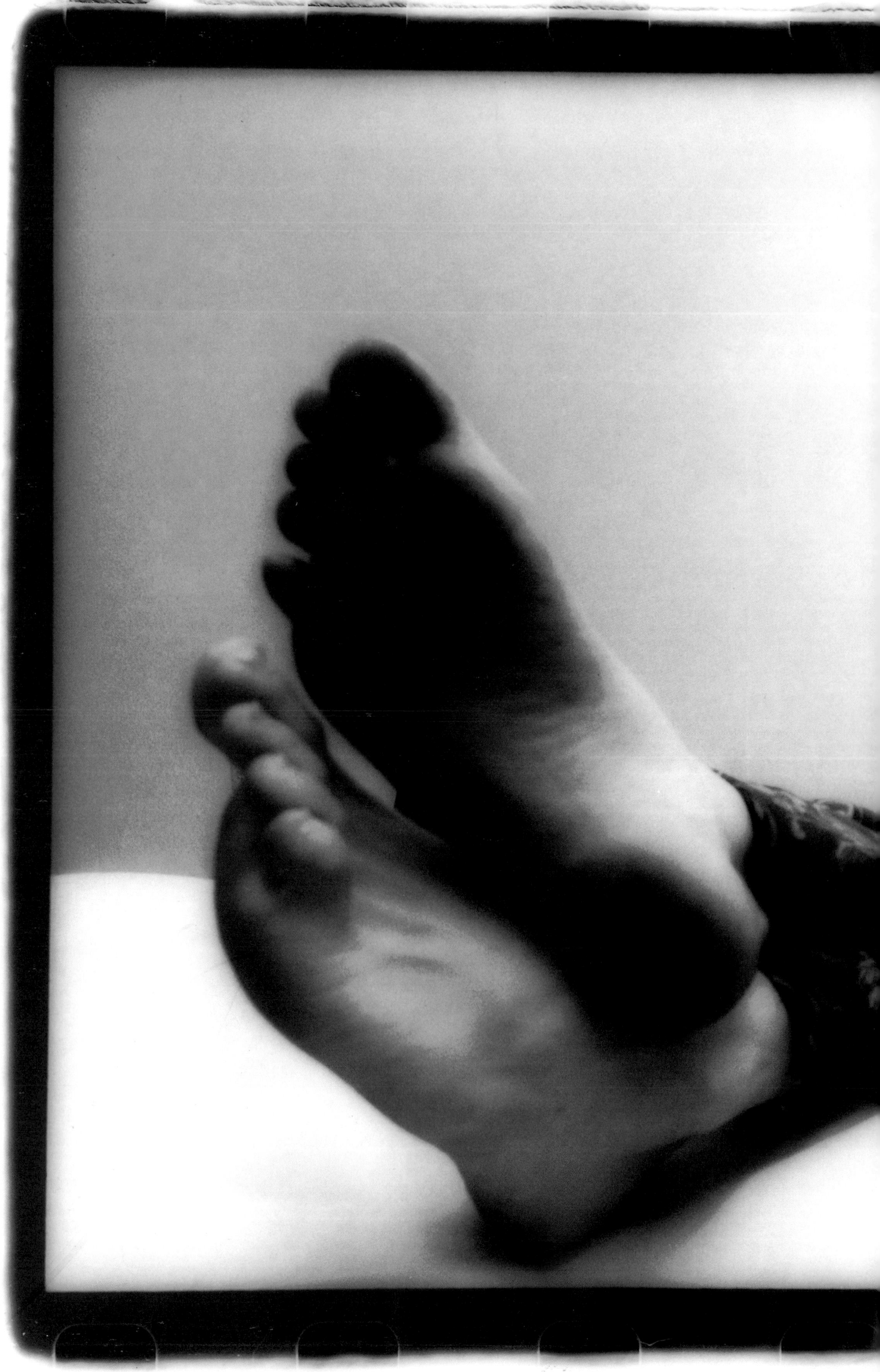

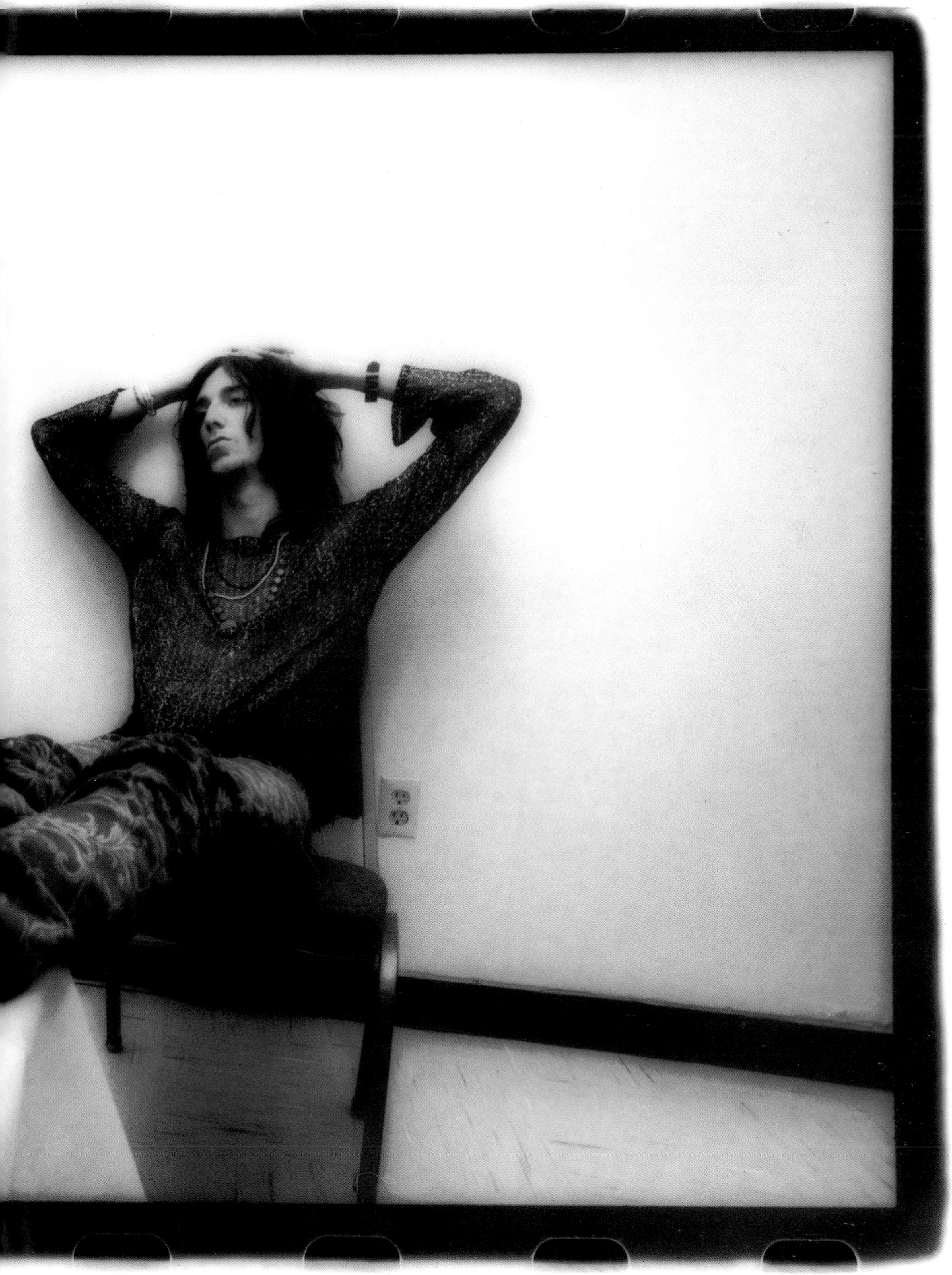

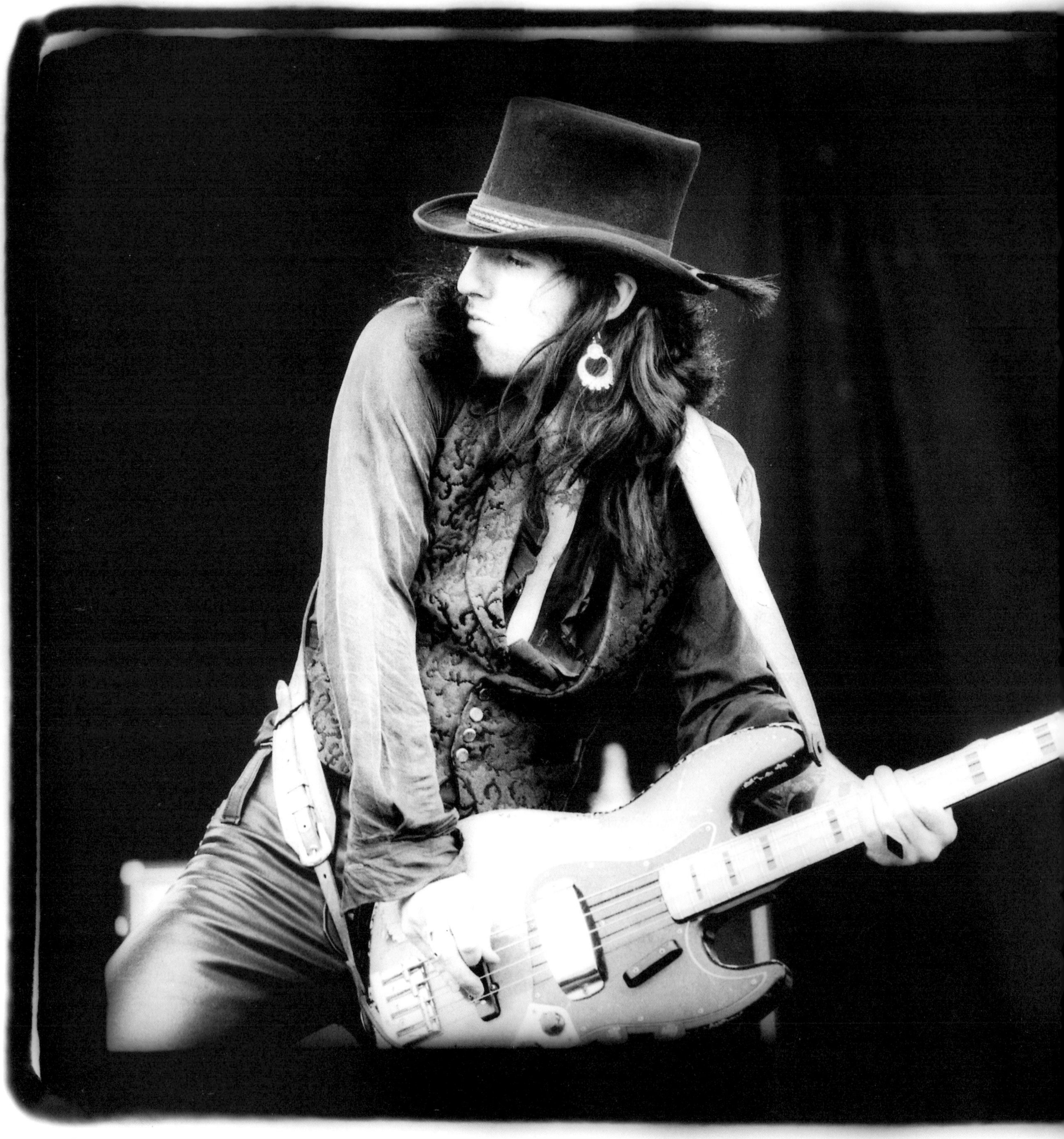

Johnny Colt

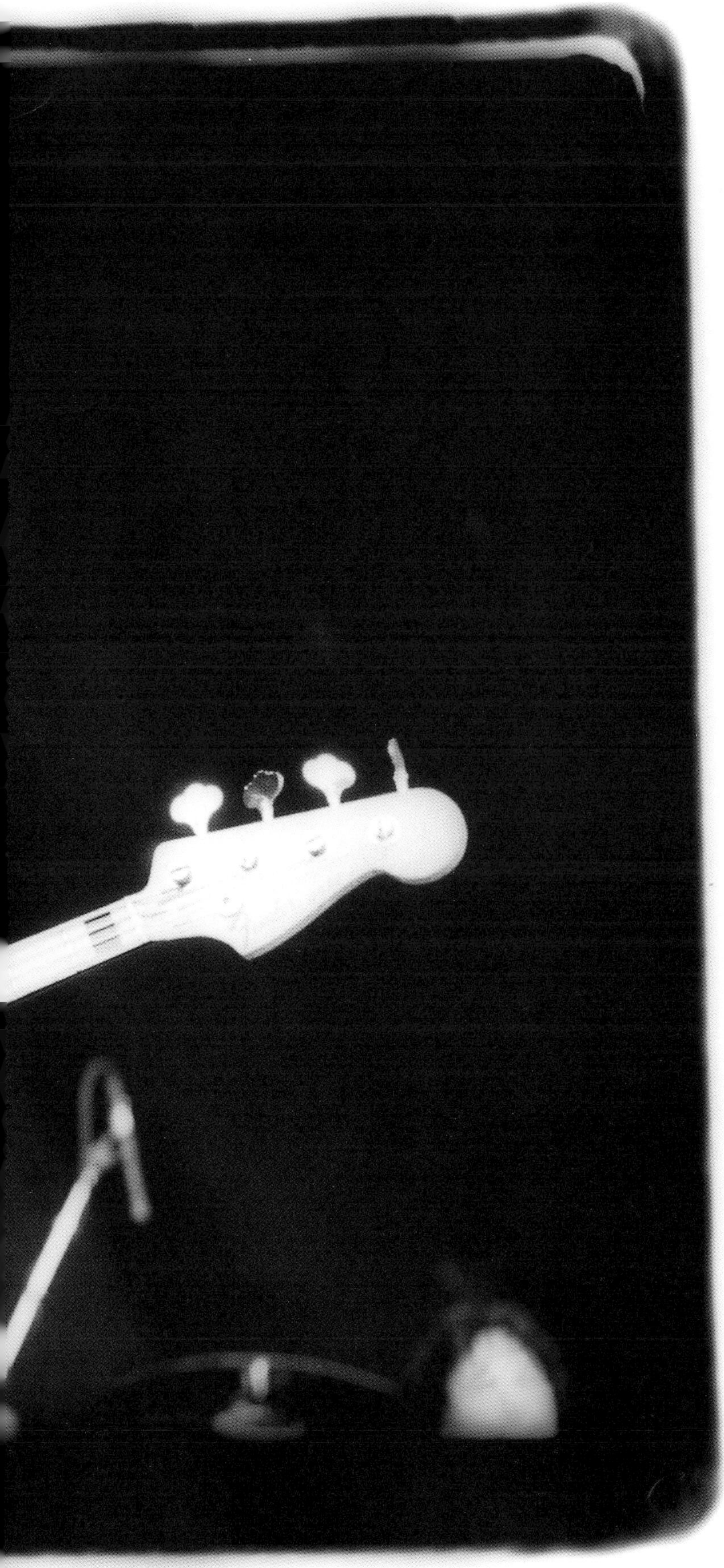

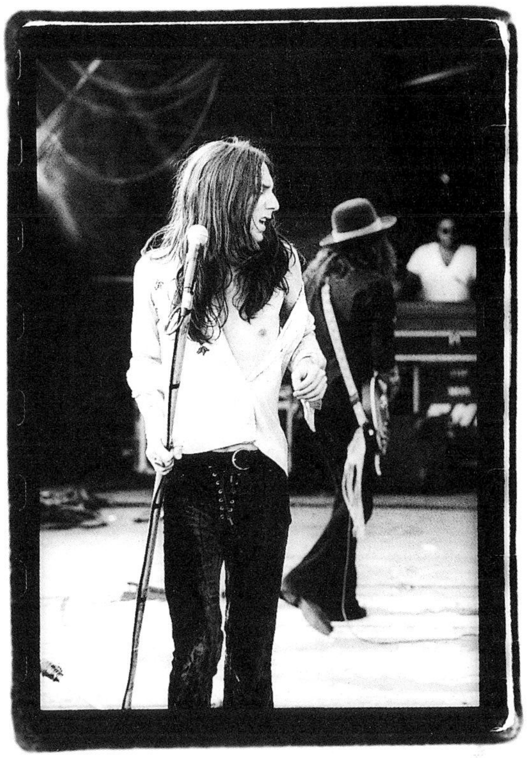

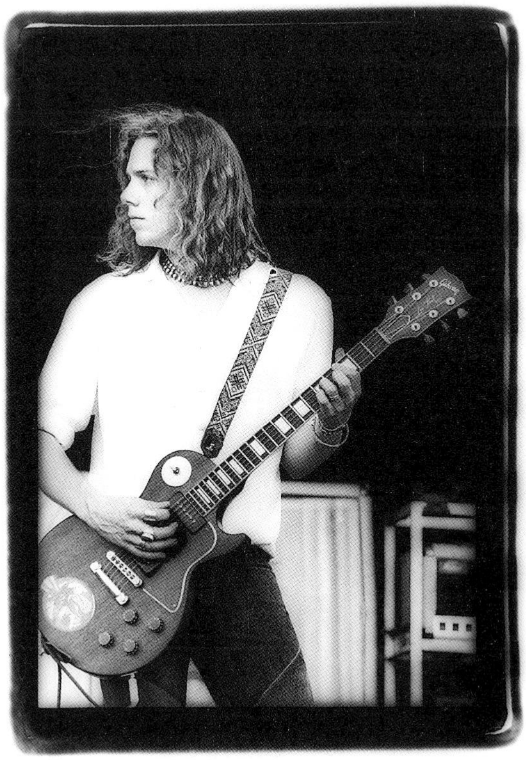

Chris And Rich Robinson
Belgium, '93

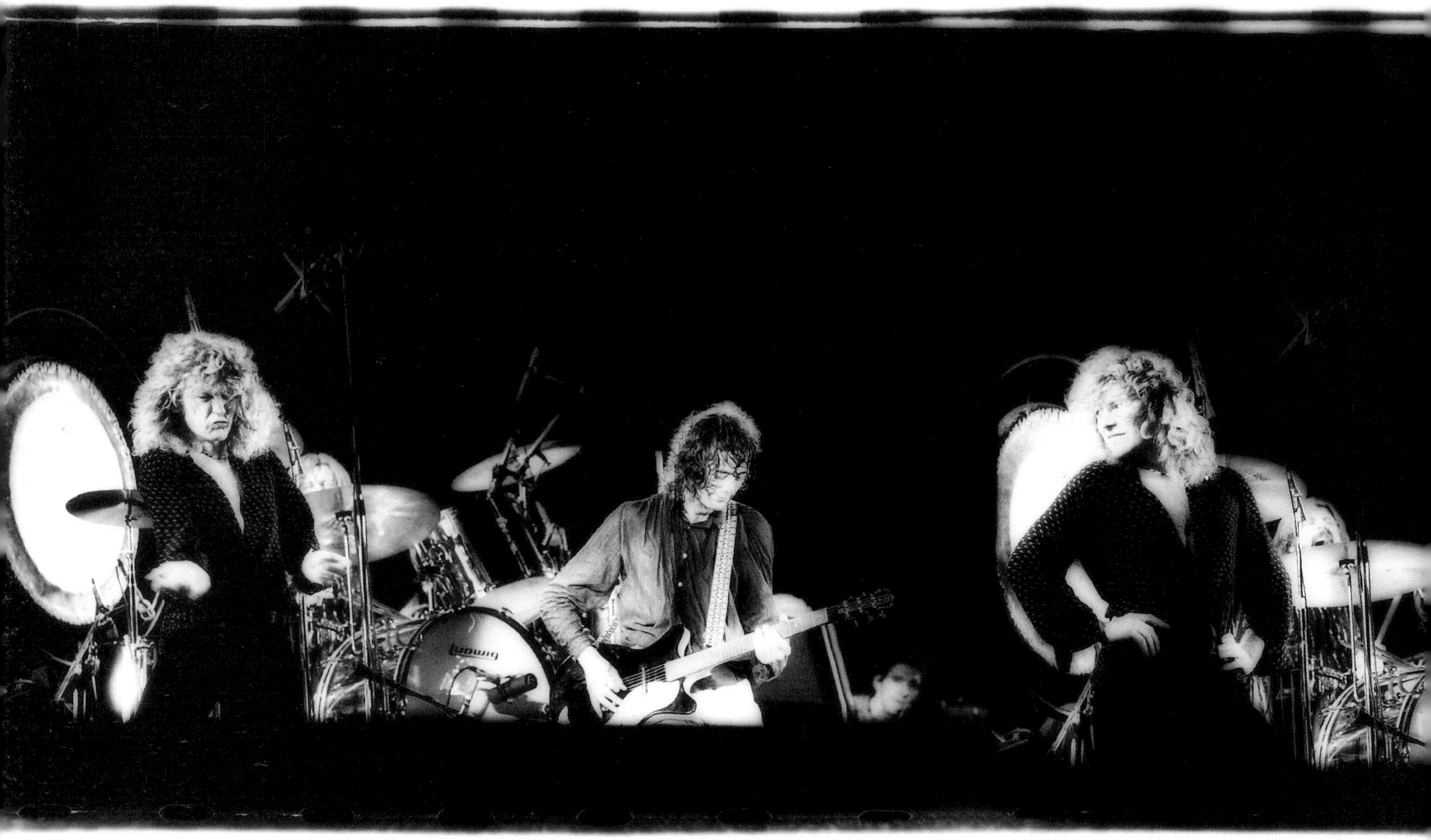

LED ZEPPELIN

I shot Led Zeppelin on August 11th, 1979 at Knebworth (which was the last time they played in England, and also happened to be my birthday). After shooting the other acts all day, Zeppelin decided that we had to shoot them from about half a mile away.

Just before they came on stage, Chalkie Davis (photographer) and I bumped into BP Fallon (Zep's PR) who was speeding out of his head. We said, rather sarcastically, "How about getting them to do a line-up shot before they go on?" And he was, like, "Oh, yeah, great, not a problem." So we were walked into the inner sanctum and Zeppelin lined up for us for about ten minutes. The only problem was that my flash gun was not set properly and all I ended up with was them from the knees down.

We were told we still couldn't shoot live, so after listening to the set from under the stage for half an hour, we decided to climb the scaffolding and ended up on the video ramp. A big American came over and screamed, "What are you doing? You can't come up here!" We told him Peter Grant had said it was OK and he let us get on with it, and we shot the last hour of the show from there.

Ross Halfin

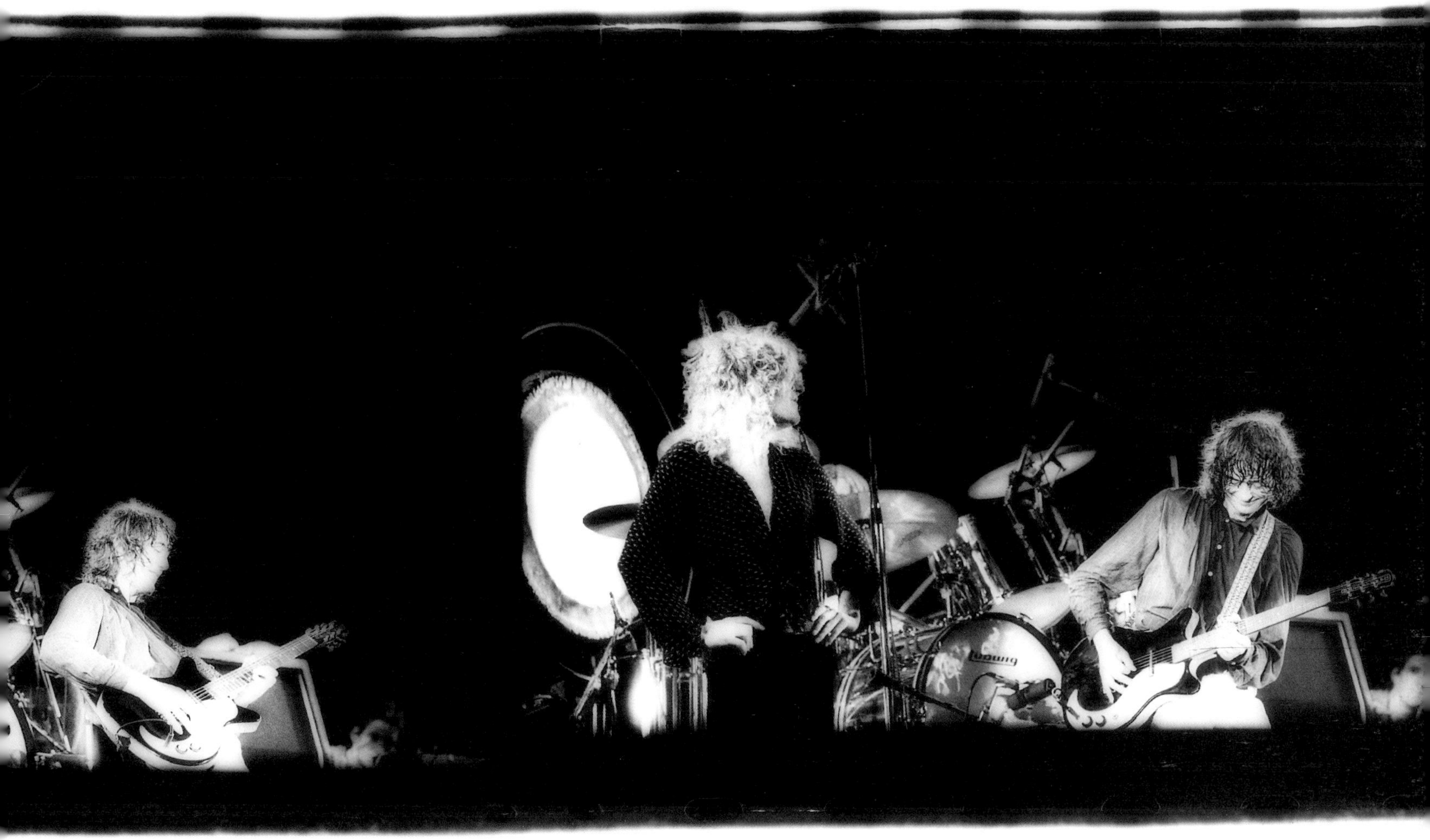

Led Zeppelin, Knebworth, August 11, 1979

robert plant

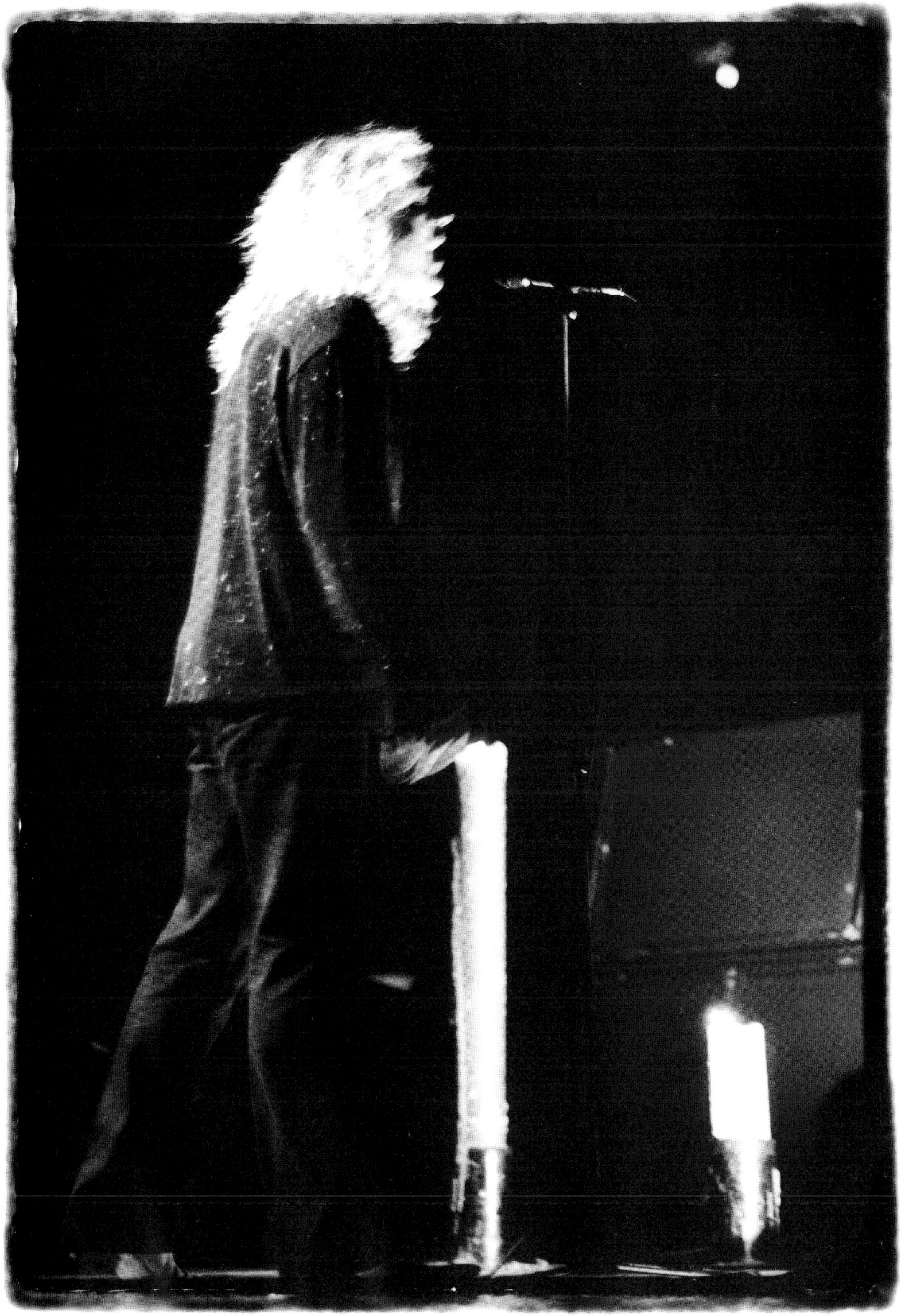

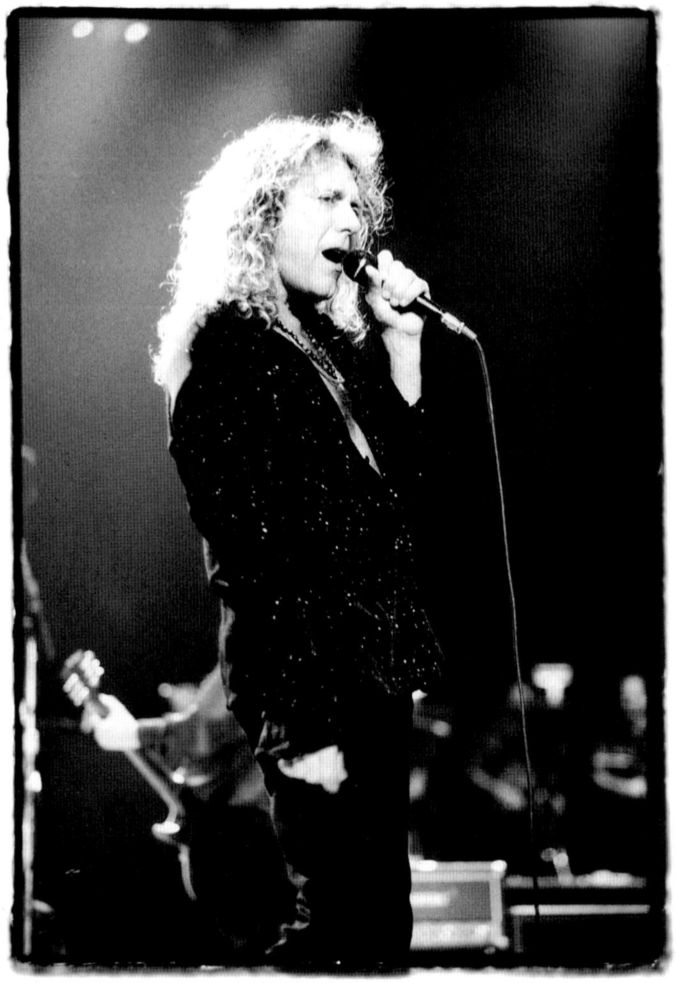

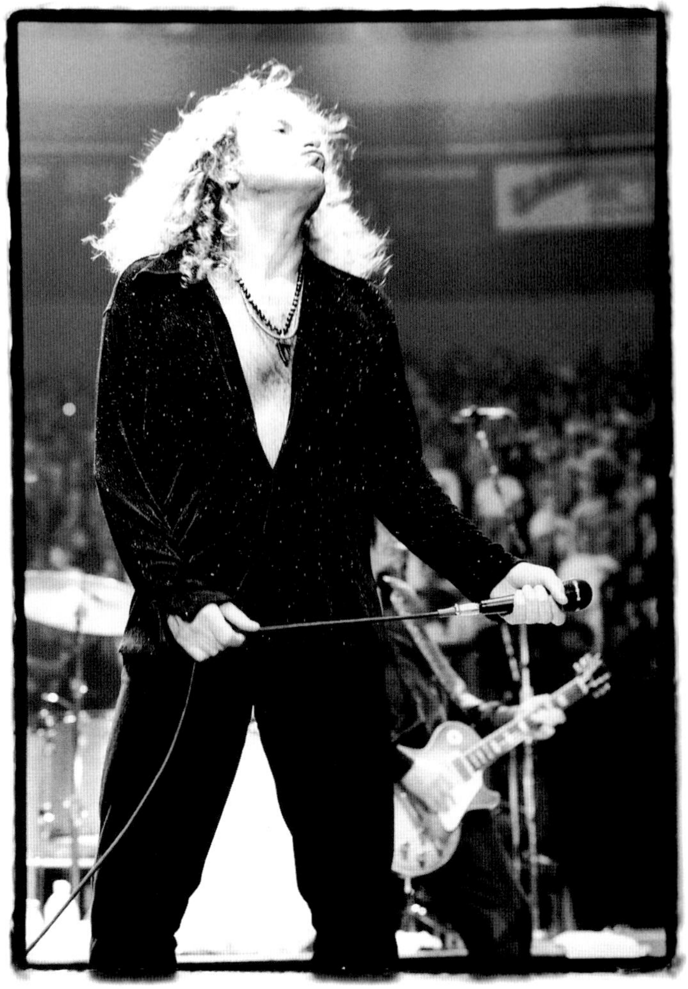

ROBERT PLANT

I shot Robert Plant solo for the first time in '83 at Blakes Hotel in London. He walked up to me with a nice big smile on his face and said, "Do you know how to take a Robert Plant picture?" Me, all polite and innocent, "Er no," so he leant in my face, poked me in the chest and said, "Quickly!" I took a really average picture of him that day and decided afterwards not to ever let anyone intimidate me again.

ROSS HALFIN

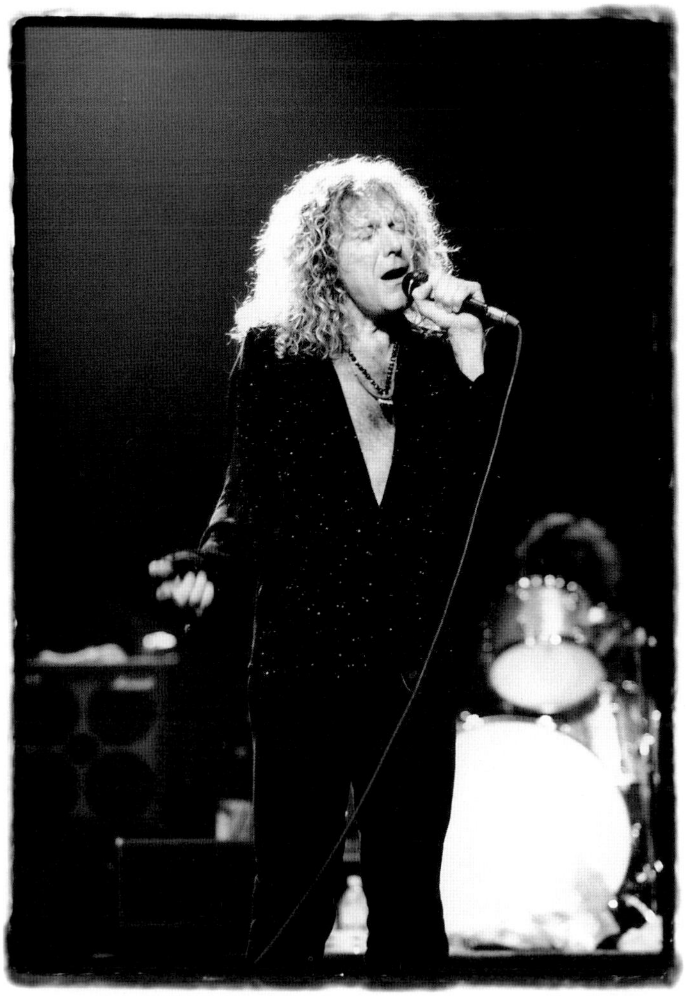

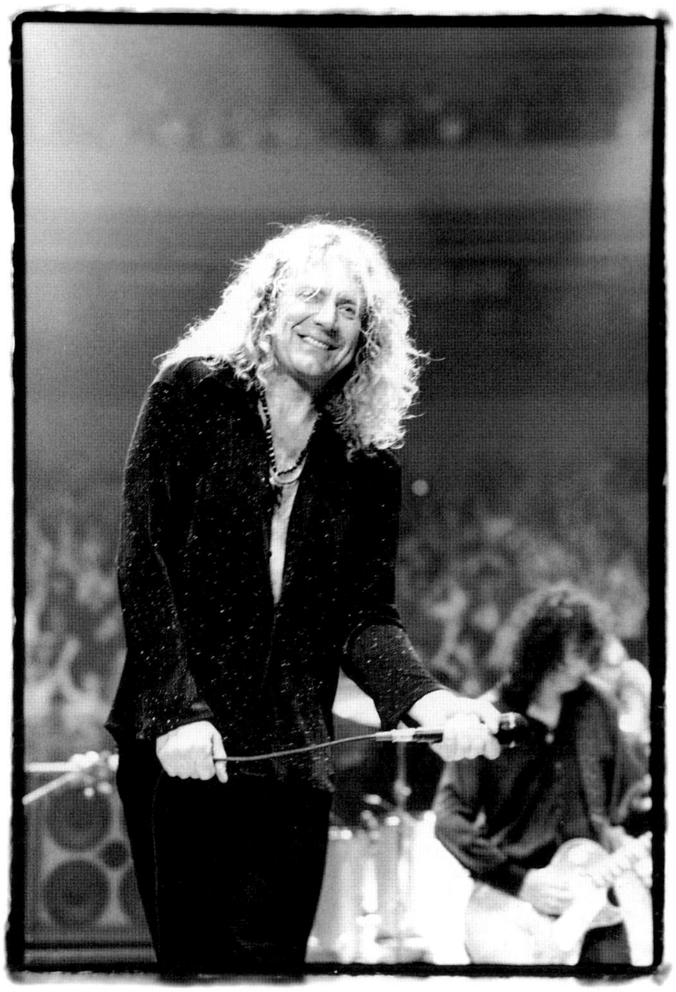

ROBERT PLANT, MADISON SQUARE GARDEN
OCTOBER 27, 1995

jimmy page

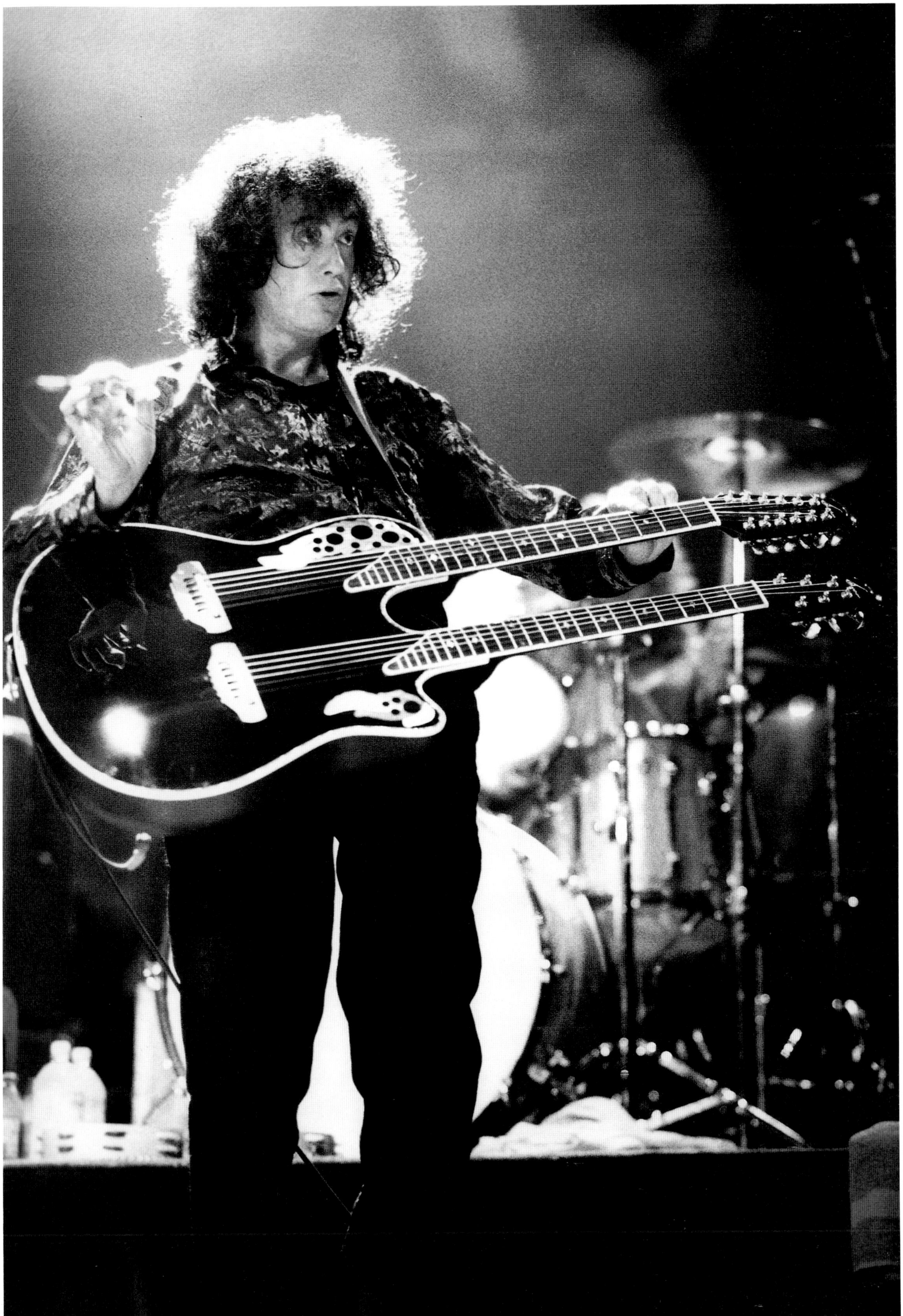

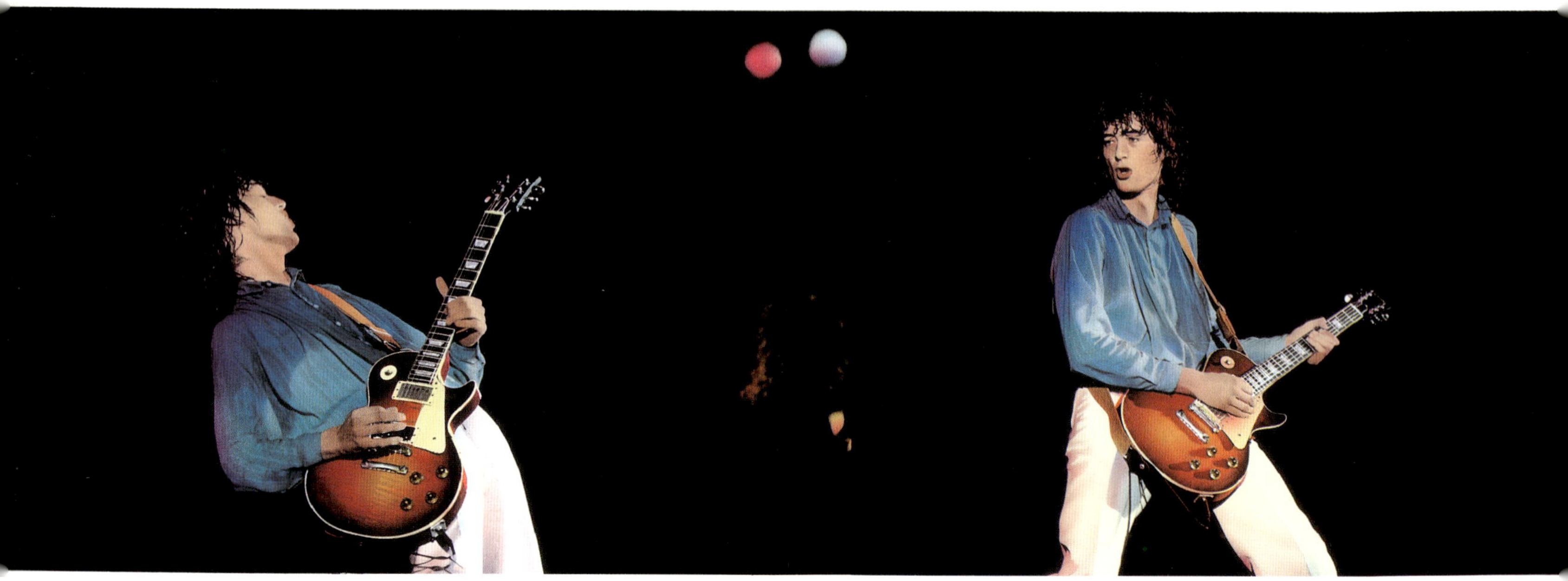

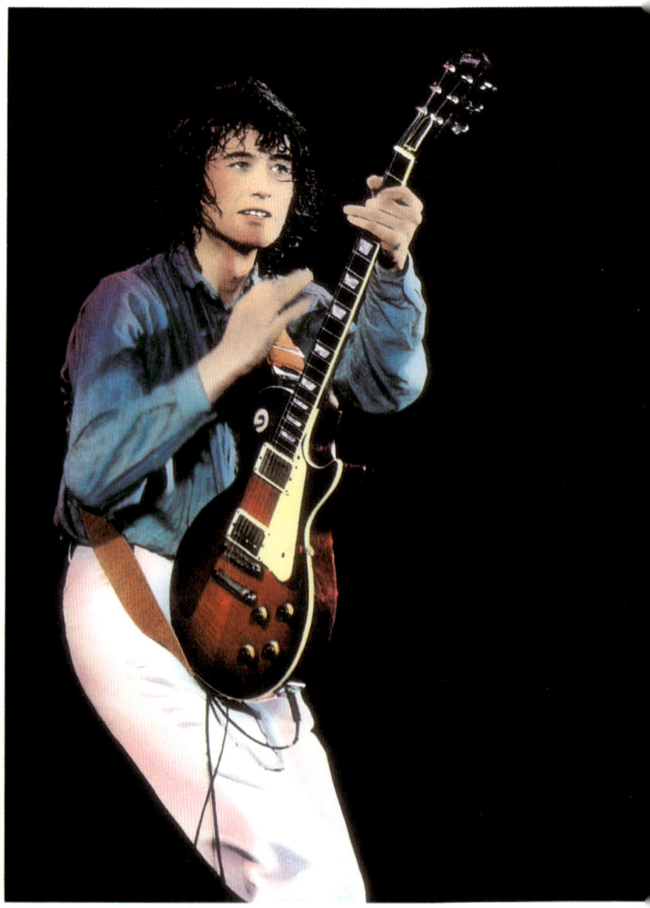

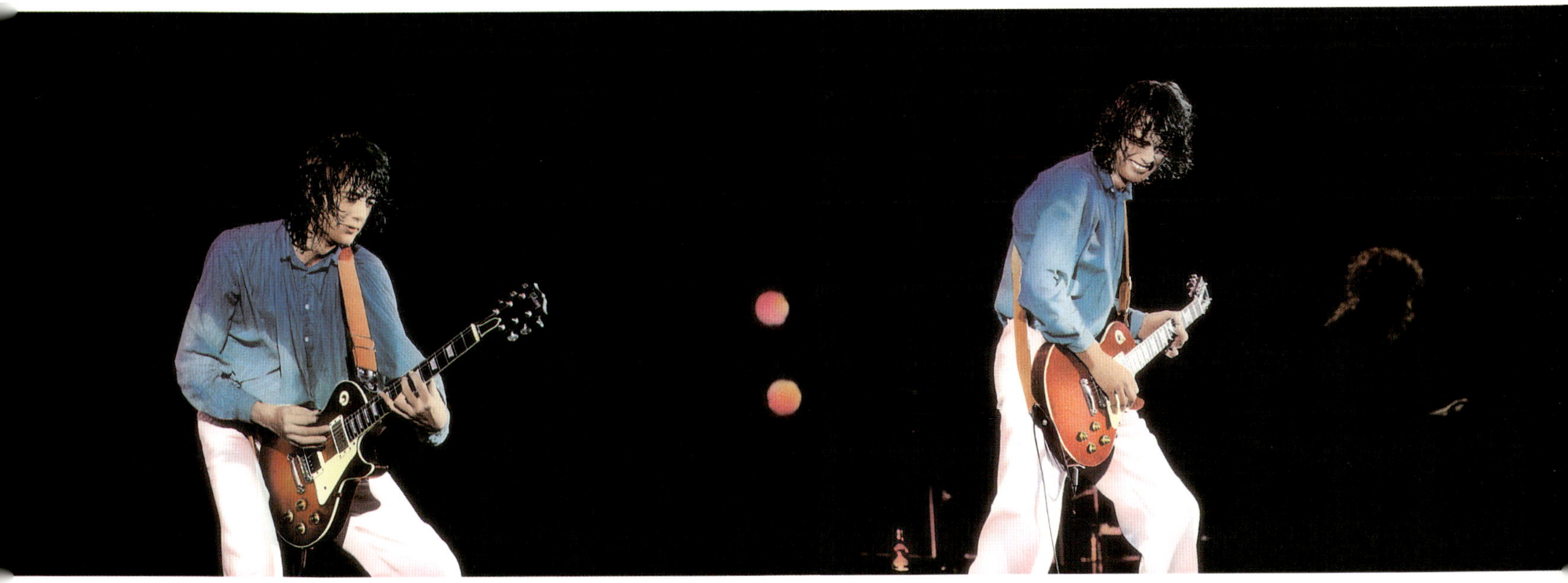

JIMMY PAGE, LIVE, KNEBWORTH, AUGUST 11, 1979

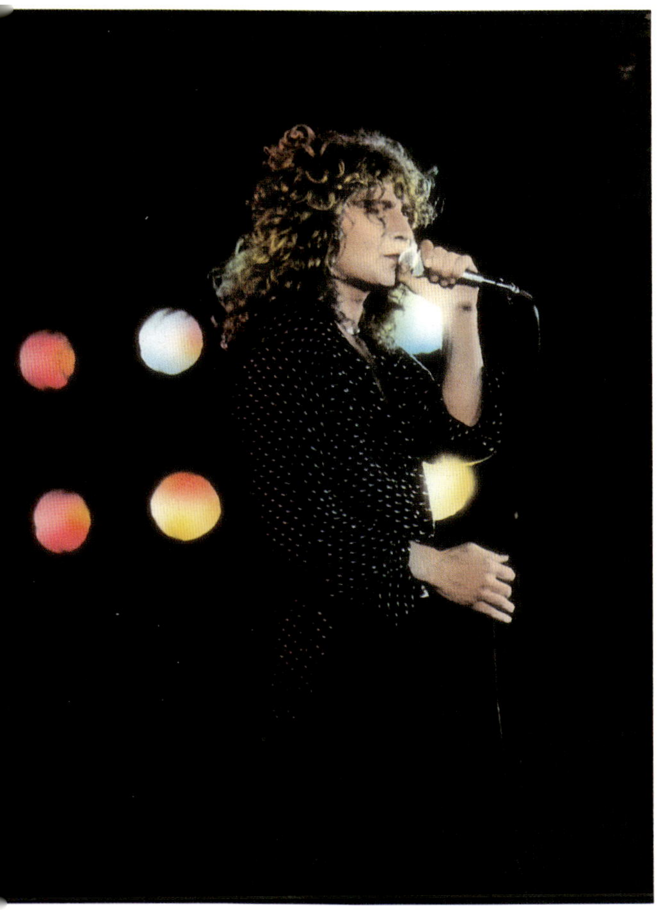

LED ZEPPELIN

I saw Led Zeppelin. The curtain went up. White lights almost blinding. Kashmir. Eighteen thousand people merely cushioned the blow. They were bigger than we were. They swallowed the place whole. If you're in a hard rock band and you're playing something good, you have to check yourself to see if you're ripping off Jimmy Page... All these boys making a living sounding like Robert Plant. Bonzo ate drums for breakfast. Zep slid through their musical styles like a hot knife through Mick Jagger. If you play their records now they're still great. Timeless.

Henry Rollins

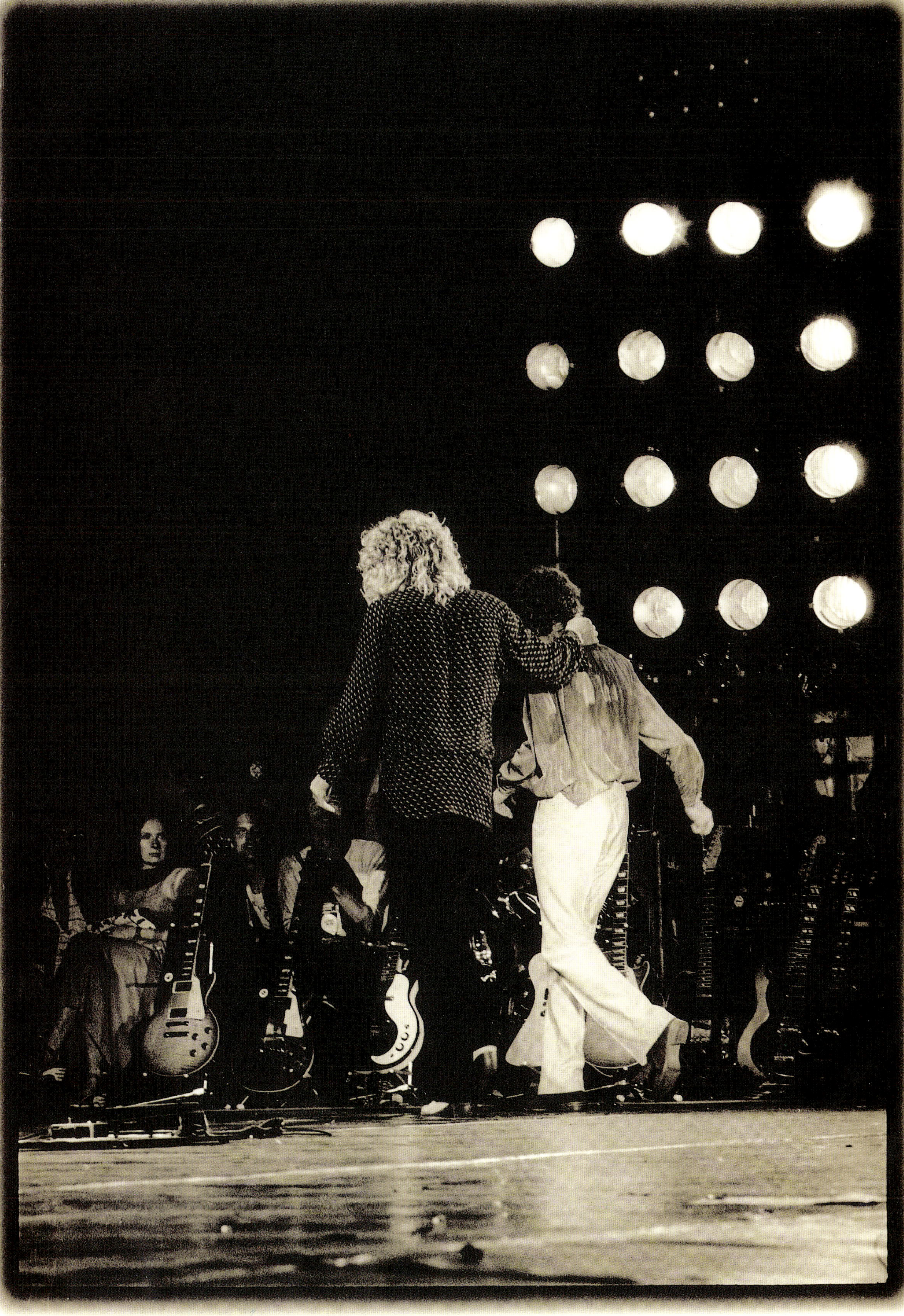

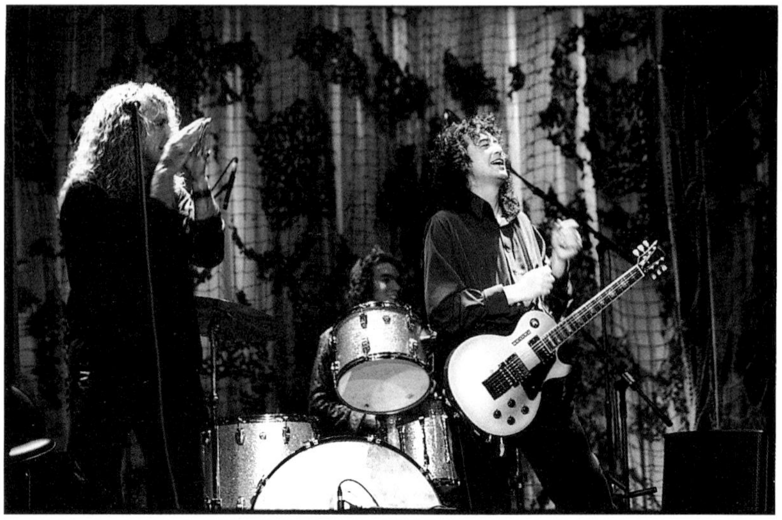

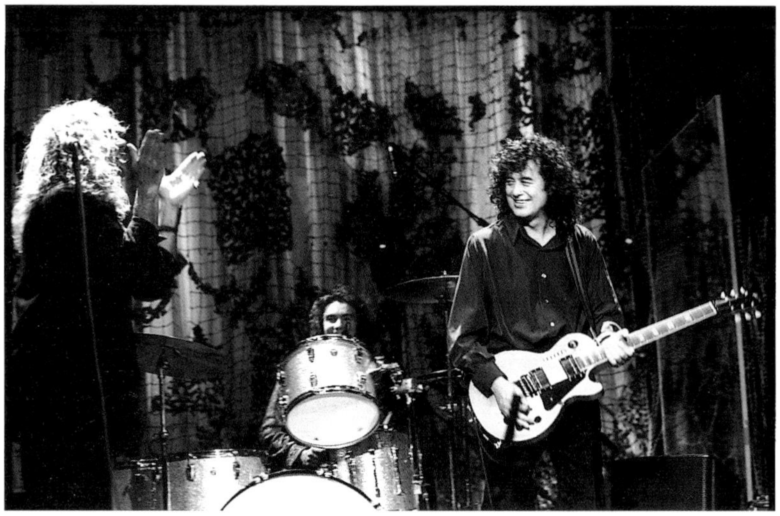

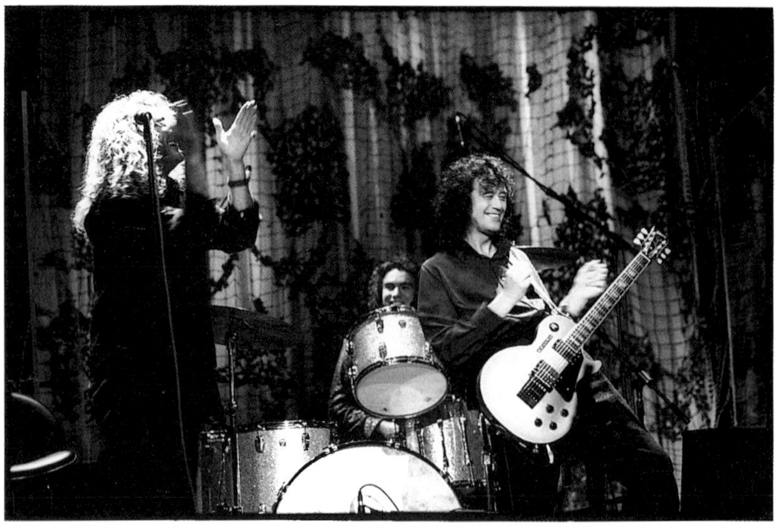

Page, Plant, Plant, Page
London
1994

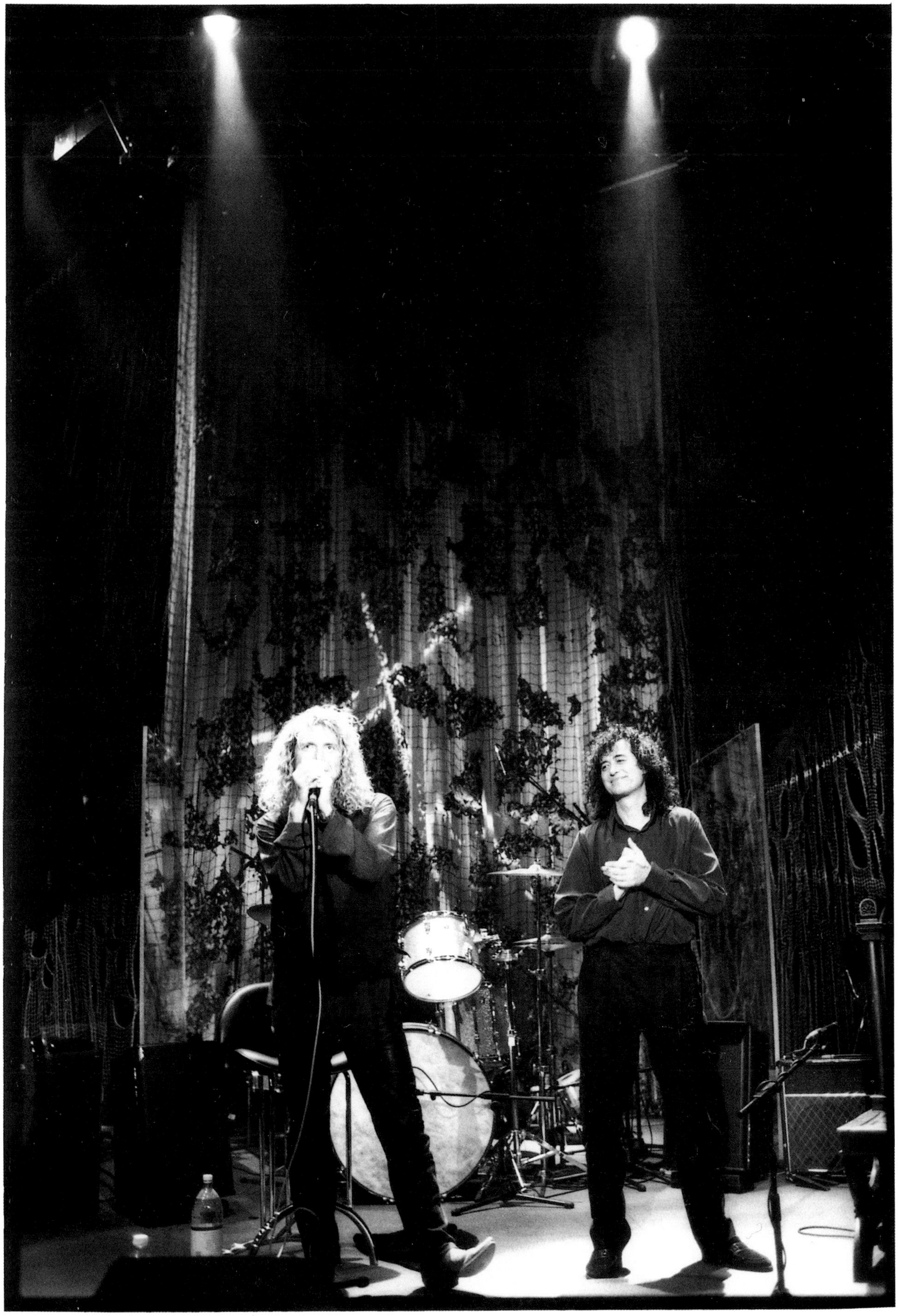

metallica

Metallica
Red Square
Moscow

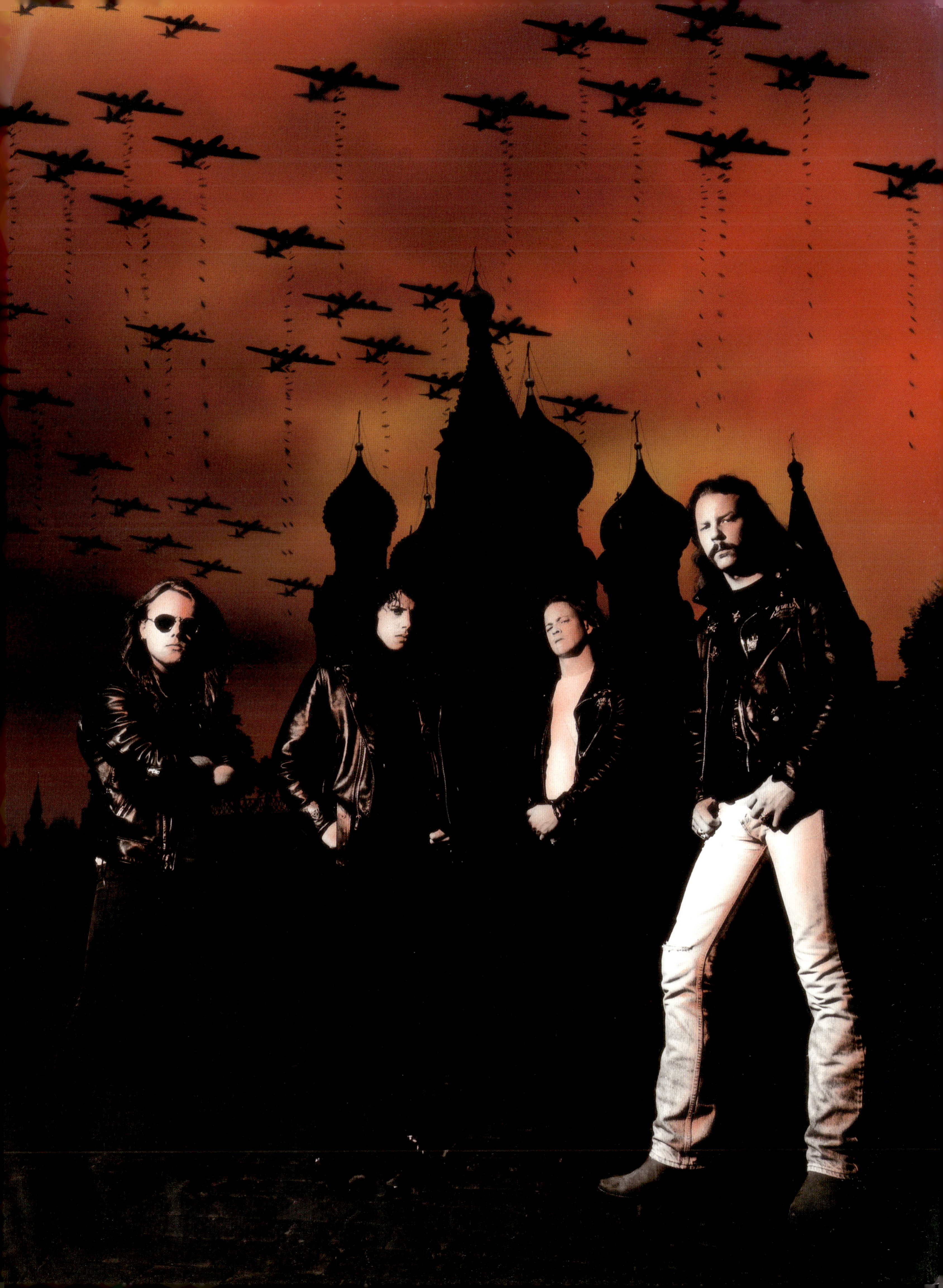

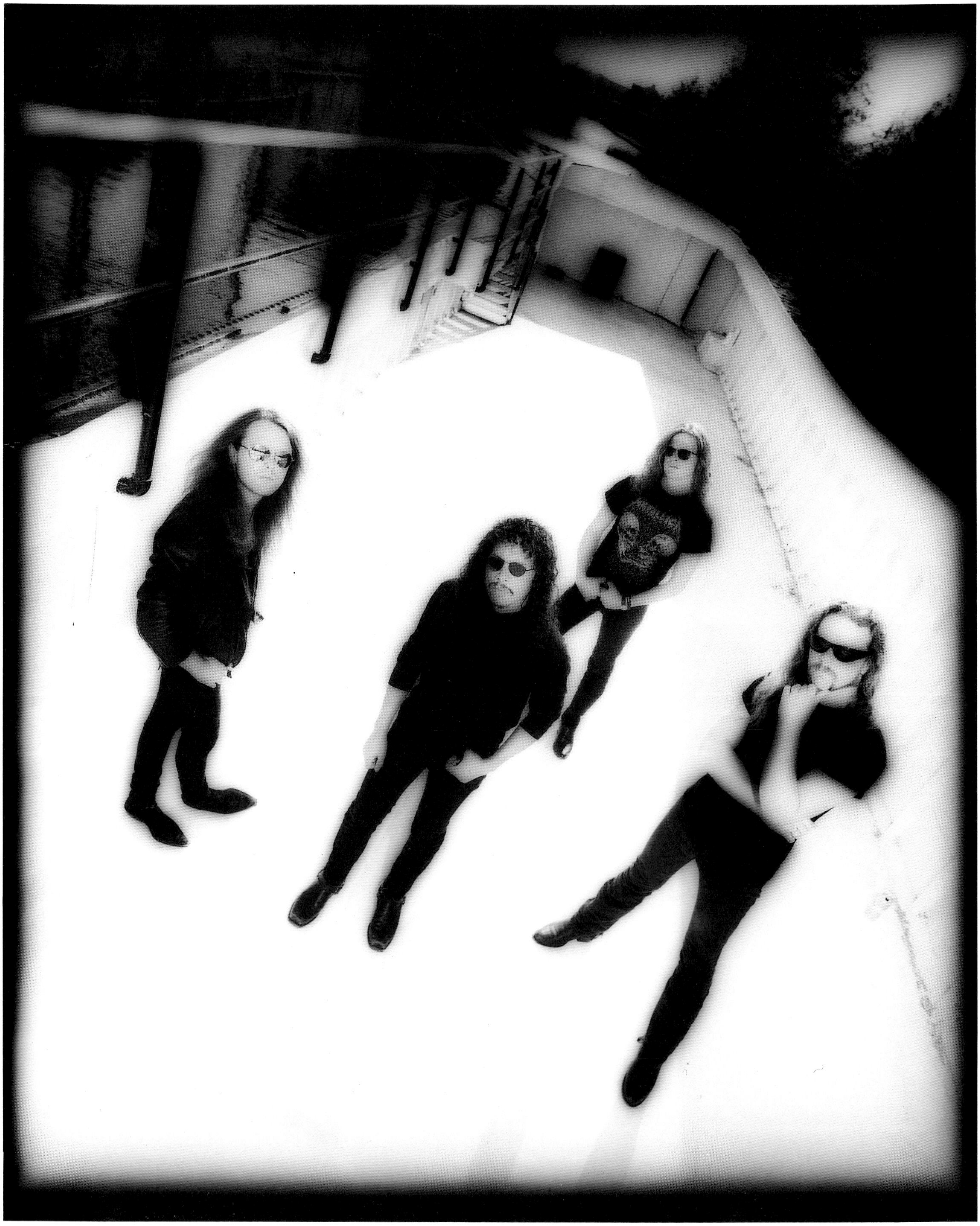

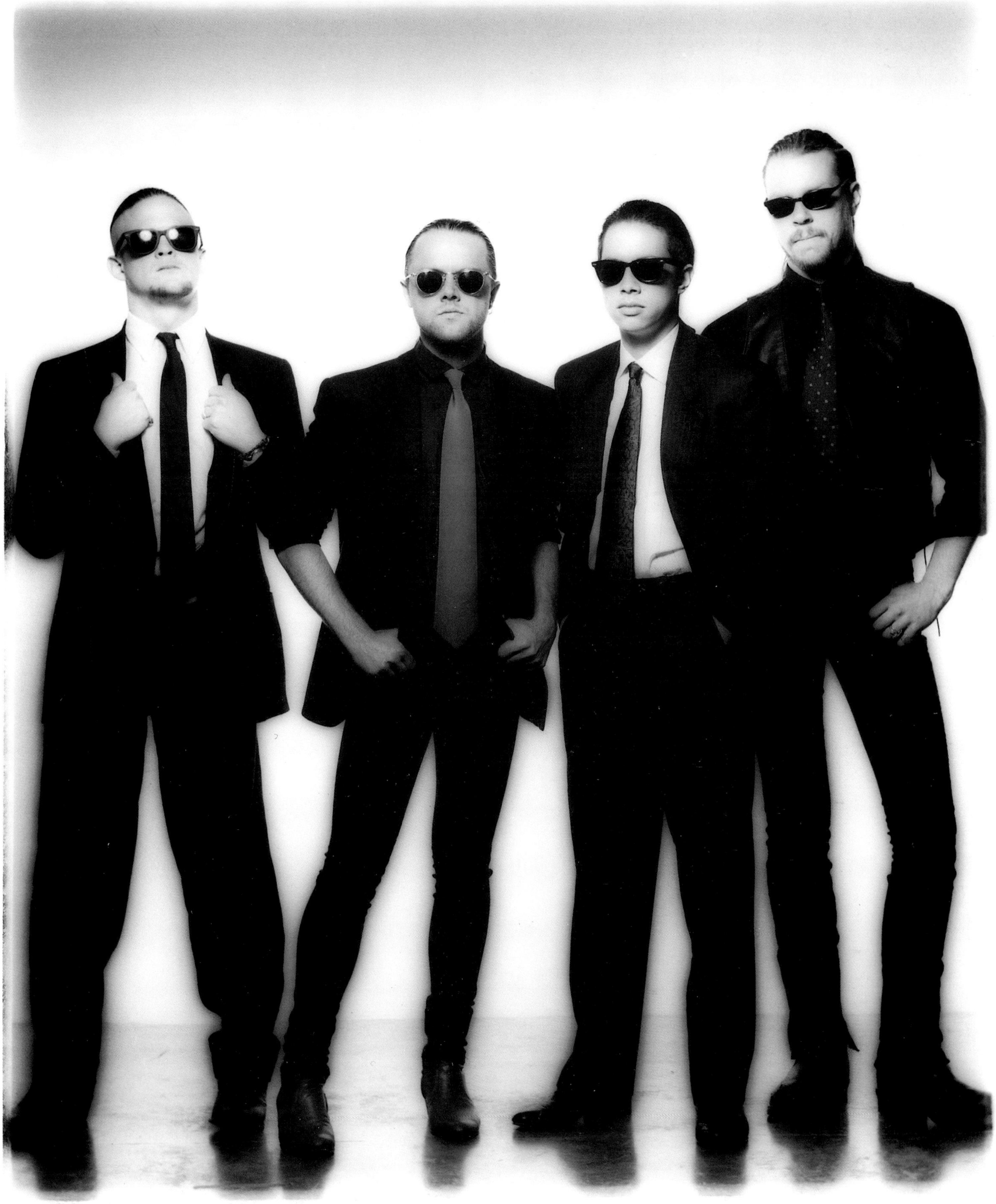

(1)

~~HAT~~

WHAT I DID ON MY SUMMER VAKATION
BY. JAYMZ HATEFIELD

DAY 1: WENT OUT TO LOOK FOR A JOB
DAY 2: WENT OUT TO LOOK FOR A JOB
ENDED UP HANGING OUT IN FRONT OF THE DRUG STORE
DAY 3-6: WENT OUT TO LOOK FOR A JOB
ENDED UP HANGING OUT IN FRONT OF THE DRUG STORE
DAY 7: GOT A JOB KEEPING KIDZ FROM HANGIN OUT
IN FRONT OF THE DRUG STORE

METALLICA TOUR: MONTH OF MAY
GOAL: SWINDLE THE PROMOTER INTO PAYING ENOUGH MONEY
FOR US TO ~~VACATION~~ PLAY IN THE LANDS DOWN UNDER.

NEW ZEALAND:
DAY 1 - UNKNOWN
4 DAYZ IN AUKLAND = PLENTY OF RAIN
PLENTY OF [redacted] THE SAME MOVIE
PLENTY OF SHEEP
PLENTY OF MUTANTS
(SHEEP OUT NUMBER MUTANTS 4-1)
PLENTY OF BEERZ !!
OH YEA ONE JOLLY SWEATY 616

AUSTRALIA [redacted] ~~MATE~~ C-YA
GIGZ: MELBOURNE, ADELAIDE, SYDNEY
SUPPORT ACT: MORTAL SIN ~~DICKS~~ KOOL GUYZ, WAYNE = NUT
GIG DAY TRAVEL BETWEEN MELBOURNE-ADELAIDE. - CHARTERED PLANE -
THE PILOT LOOKED SUSPECT WHEN HE WALKED ON THE PLANE WITH A BAGGY CONTAINING A WHITE FLUFFY SUBSTANCE AND A LARGE BOTTLE OF RED WINE. HALF WAY THROUGH 1½ HOUR FLIGHT FOUND THE PILOT RADIOING IN HIS LAST WILL AND TESTAMENT ALSO ASSURING US THAT EVERYTHING IS O.K. (ALSO LAST THING HEARD ON [redacted] BUDDY HOLLY AIRLINES) HES LANDED THE PLANE BEFORE WITH ONE FLAMING ENGINE [redacted]

(2)

INFLIGHT QUOTES:
"I CANT DIE, I HAVENT SEEN MY RE-MODELED KITCHEN YET" - P. MENCH
"OH PLEASE DONT LET US DIE PLEASE DONT LET US DIE I WONT SAY THE WORD SATAN EVER AGAIN" - K. HAMMETT
RECITING LYRICS TO HIS FAVORITE WASP SONG - L. ULRICH
LISTENING TO NAT KING COLE C.D. - J. NEWKID
"AAAAHH HOW DO YOU OPEN THIS DOOR" - R. HALFAN (PHOTOGRAFER(?))
"WHAT ABOUT THE KIDZ?" - [redacted] T. DIGIOCCO (ACCOUNTANT & BUD)
"THIS IS NOT A WIND-UP" - B. SCHNEIDER (TOUR MANAGER, LOUD VOICE)
"ZZZZZ ZZZZZZZZ" [redacted] T. SMITH (ASSISTANT BEER FETCHER)

AFTER GIG DID A RUNNER BACK TO MELBOURNE BECAUSE A CERTAIN BAND MEMBER'S WIFE WAS OUT (HINT: K-RK)

SYDNEY: PHOTO SHOOTS
DAY 1 - LARZ'S HIGHLY ORIGINAL & BRILLIANT IDEA TO SHOOT IN FRONT OF SYDNEY OPERA HOUSE.
DAY 2 - LARZ: "HEY LETS SHOOT IN FRONT OF THE OPERA HOUSE TO MAKE SHURE ~~WE~~ GOT IT."
DAY 3 - LARZ: "WHAT ABOUT THE OPERA HOUSE?"
7 BORING HOURS LATER: "WHAT ABOUT THIS CAVE NEXT TO THE OPERA HOUSE?"

GIG IN SYDNEY:
PAT CA$H THE VERRY VERRY FAMOUS (EVEN MORE FAMOUS THAN US!) BADMINTON STAR SHOWED UP. EXTREME GROVELING GOING ON BY UNKNOWN BAND MEMBER WHO PLAYS TENNIS. ~~THE~~
THE GIGZ IN STRALIA WENT GREAT ([redacted]). HOT SWEATY SAUNA HALLZ. LOUD FUKERZ WITH WIERD ACCENTS.

JAPAN
GIGZ: 3 TOKYO, 2 OSAKA, 1 NAGOYA
[redacted] NITES OFF AT THE LEXINGTON QUEEN BAR & SHIT DANCE MUSIK WHERE [redacted] FAMOUS BASS PLAYERS HANG OUT AND MINGLE & DANCE LIKE THE BROTHAZ
FREE DRINKS IF YOU MENSION ~~YOU HAVE A GUN~~ RICHIE BLACKMORE
THROWN OUT IF YOU MENSION ROSS HALFIN
2 CREW MEMBERZ BIRTHDAYZ, ANDY (EPILEPTIC FALIDAMITE DANCER) BATTYE AND TOMMY (2 FINGERZ OF RYE) BOOTH RAGING OUT OF CONTROL

~~HAT~~

THE PLAZA
Osaka
2-2-49, Oyodo-Minami, Kita-ku, Osaka 531, Japan
PHONE: 06-453-1111 FACSIMILE: 06-454-0169 TELEX: 5245557 PLAOSA J CABLE: PLAZAHOTEL OSAKA

(3)

AT THE LEX, GETTING CLOSE TO RELIVING THE DAYZ OF EDDY THE BATHROOM BARTENDER (DONT ASK)
ANOTHER BRILLIANT IDEA OF DOING A FOTO SESSION AT THE MAIN TRAIN STATION RITE AFTER THE GIG CAUSING A MINOR RIOT, WITH TAK (PROMOTOR REP.) SHOWING US SOME OF HIZ NEW KUNG FU TECNIQUES ON THE FANZ, JUST ESCAPING AS WE WATCHED ROSS GET TRAMPLED AND CAMERA EQUIPMENT STOLEN.
WHILE IN JAPAN RECIEVED TRUCK LOADZ OF HIGHLY USEFUL GIFTS FROM THE FANZ (KITTEN TOOTHBRUSHES, SNOOPY TOWELZ, TELEPHONE LOCKS, PICTURES OF YOURSELF [redacted] STUMBLEING DRUNK INTO THE HOTEL FROM THE NITE BEFORE). BUT ITS THE THOUGHT, RITE?
EVERYONES FARTS SMELL DIFFERENT, TO MUCH SUSHI.
A CERTAIN BAND MEMBER SHITS HIS PANTS DURING PHOTO SHOOT NAMED LARZ
THE CROWDZ ARE POLITE BUT FUKING LOUD SINGING ALL THE LYRIKS TO SUCH HITS AS "LIDE THE LIGHTNING", "LAST CALLESS", "BLEADFAN" AND THE FAVORITE "CLEEPING DEATH".
WE ALWAYS HAVE HUGE AMOUNTS OF FUN IN JAPAN FOODZ GREAT DRINK SAKE BEER MACHINES ON THE STREETS.
AUSTRALIA & NEW ZEALAND WERE HAPPENIN [redacted] MEETING NEW PEOPLES FRIENDS IN NEW PLACES HOPEFULLY IT WILL BE SUMMER NEXT TIME
NOW ITS OF TO HAWAII FOR SOME WORK HA!

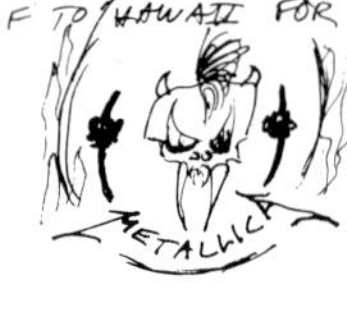

C-YA
JAYMZ

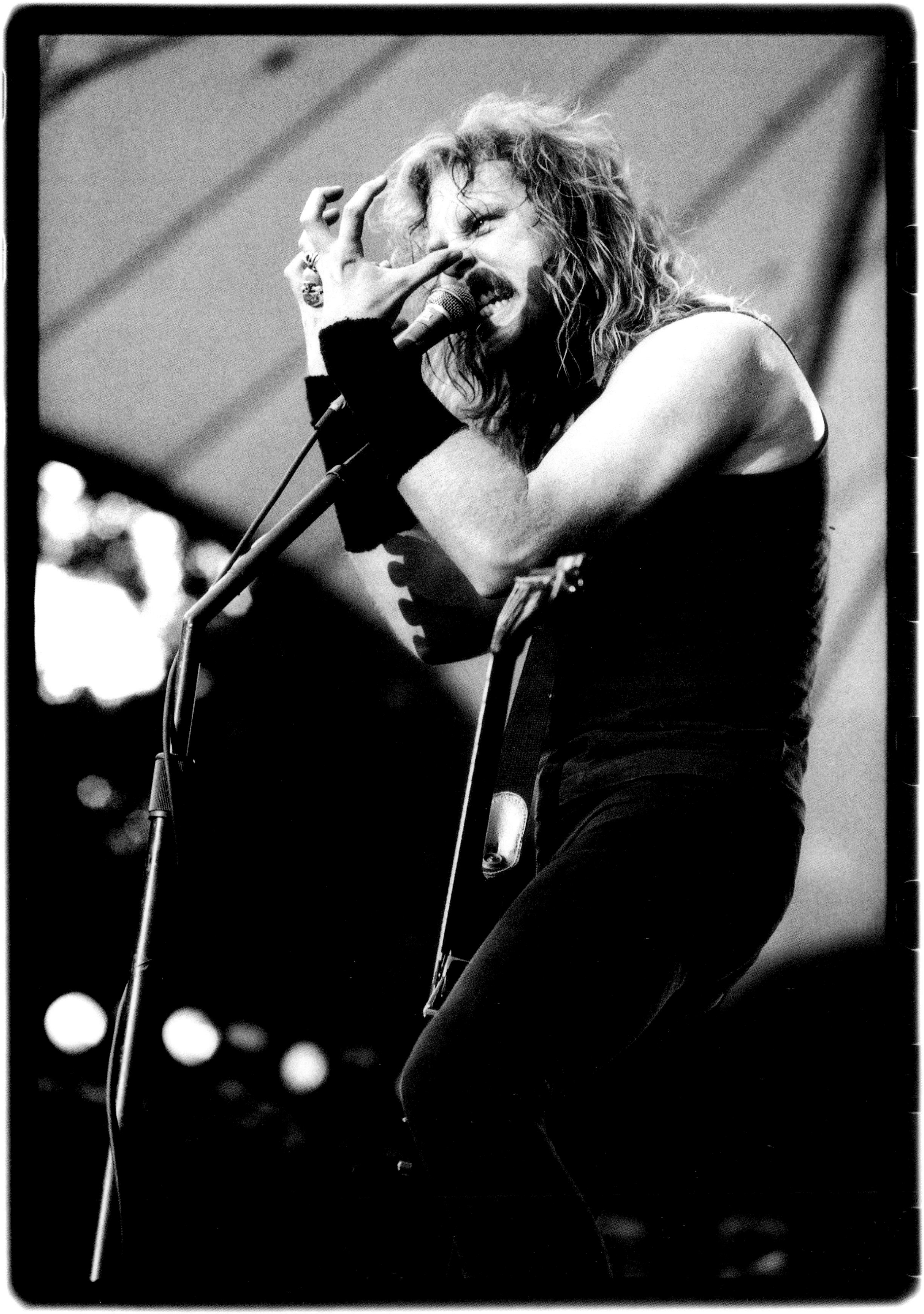

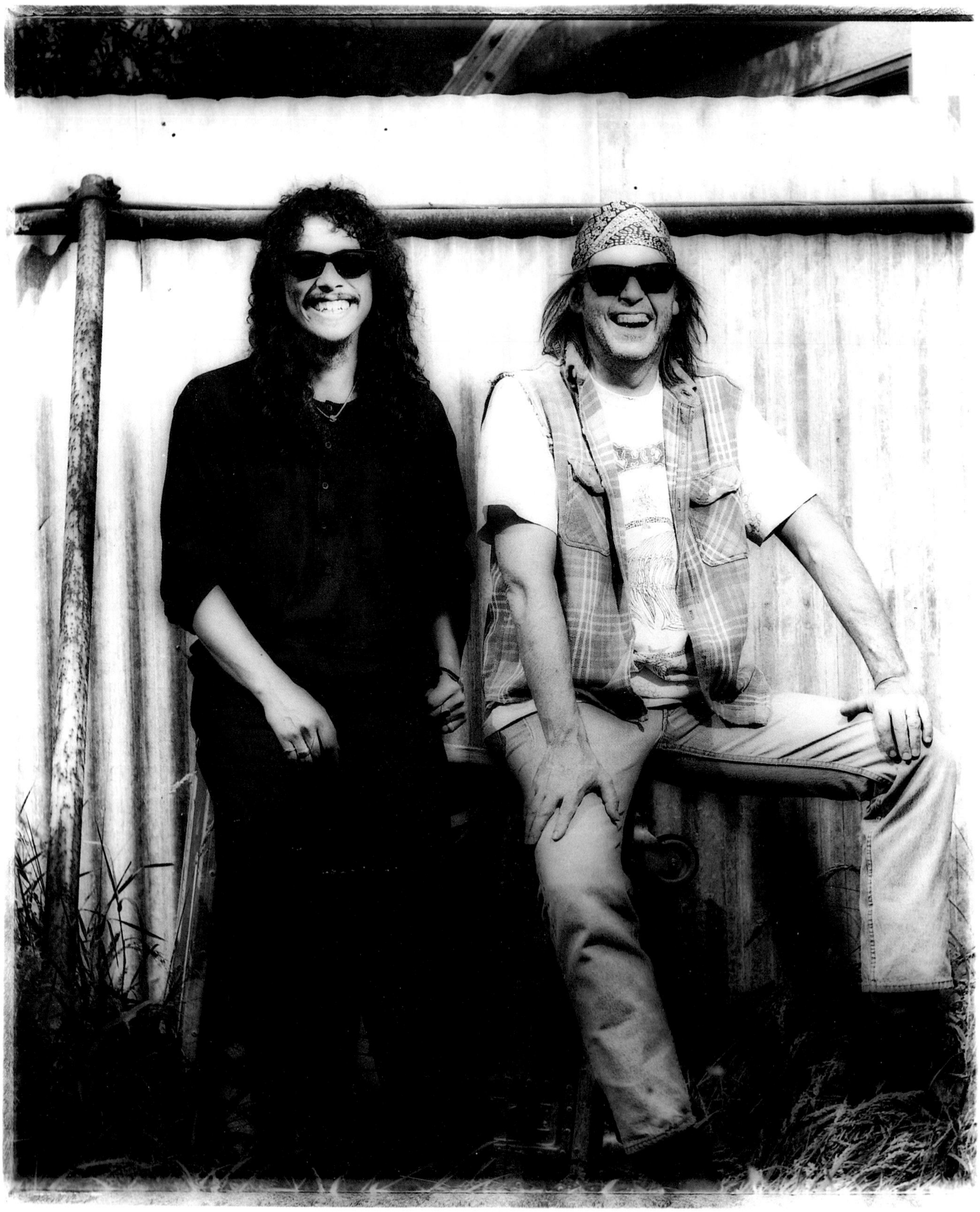

Kirk Hammett And Neil Young

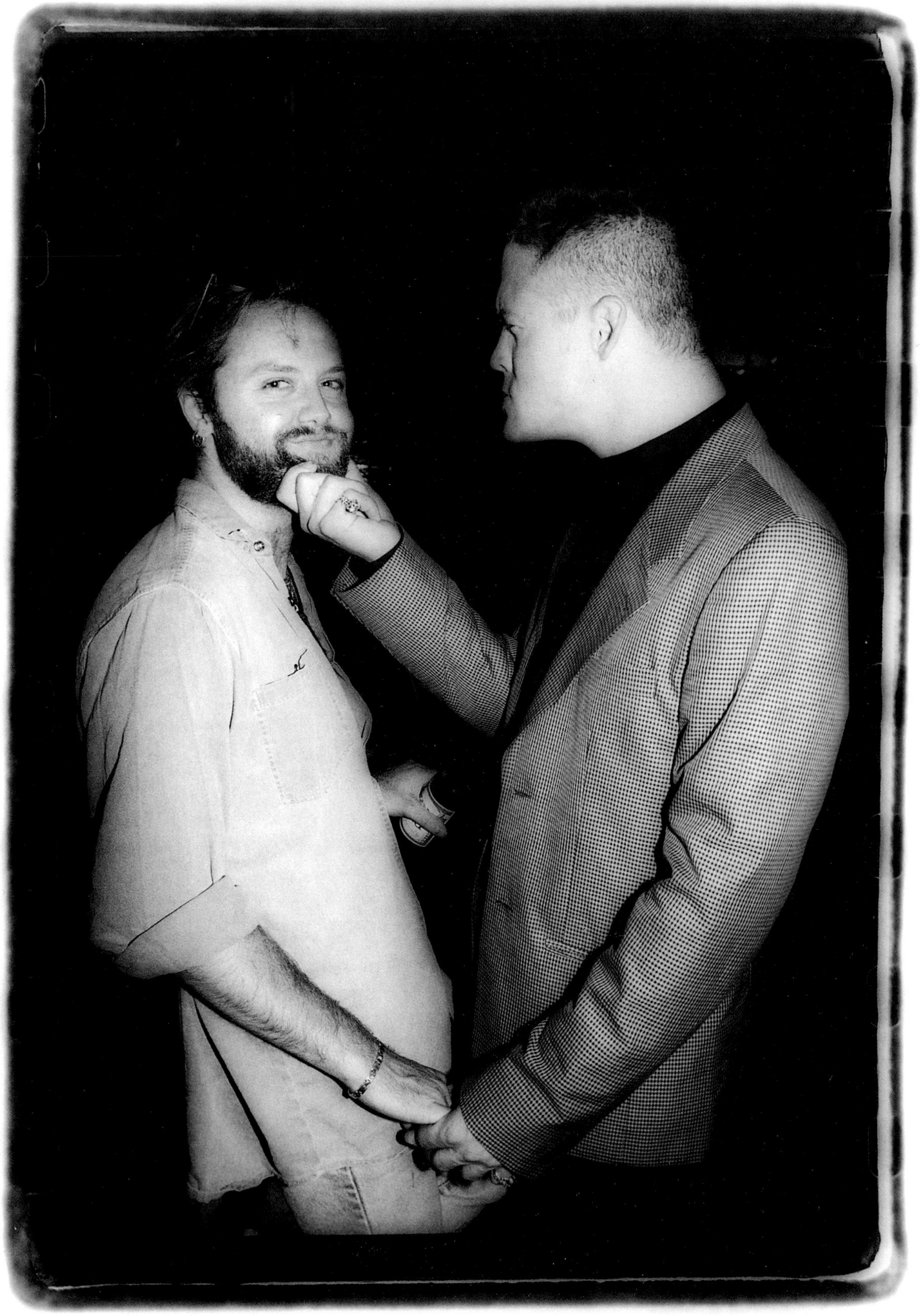

Lars And Jason

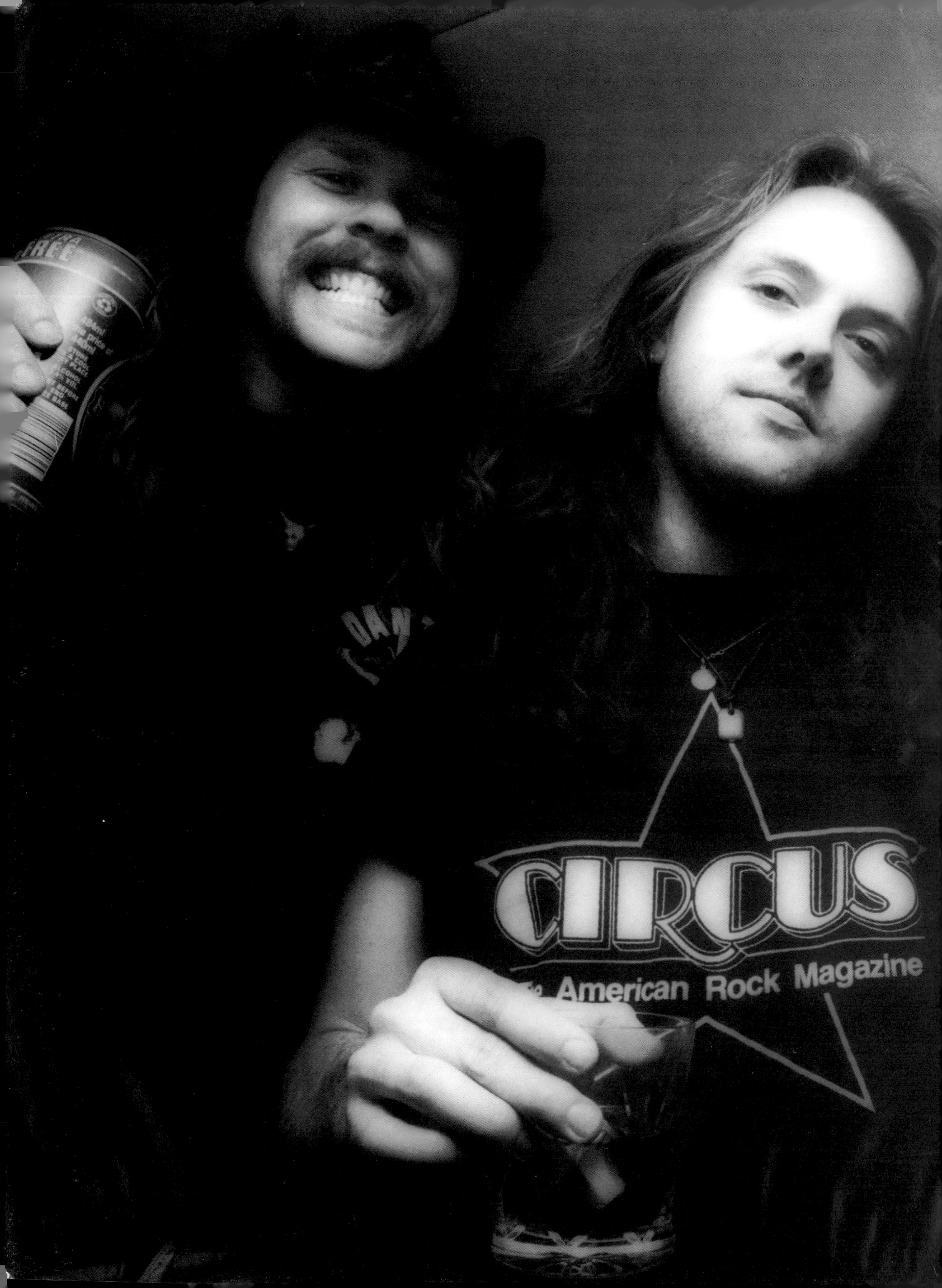
CIRCUS
American Rock Magazine

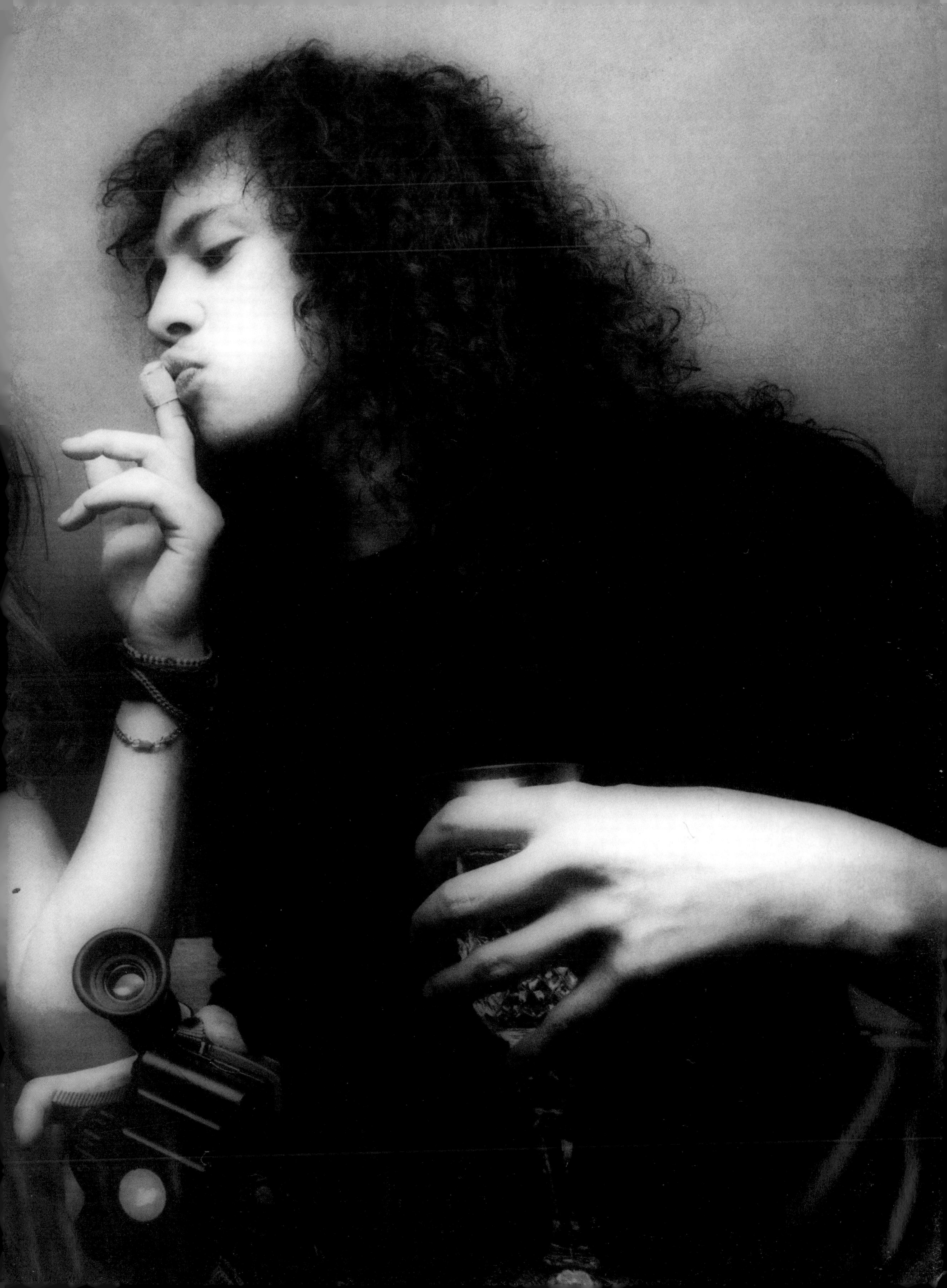

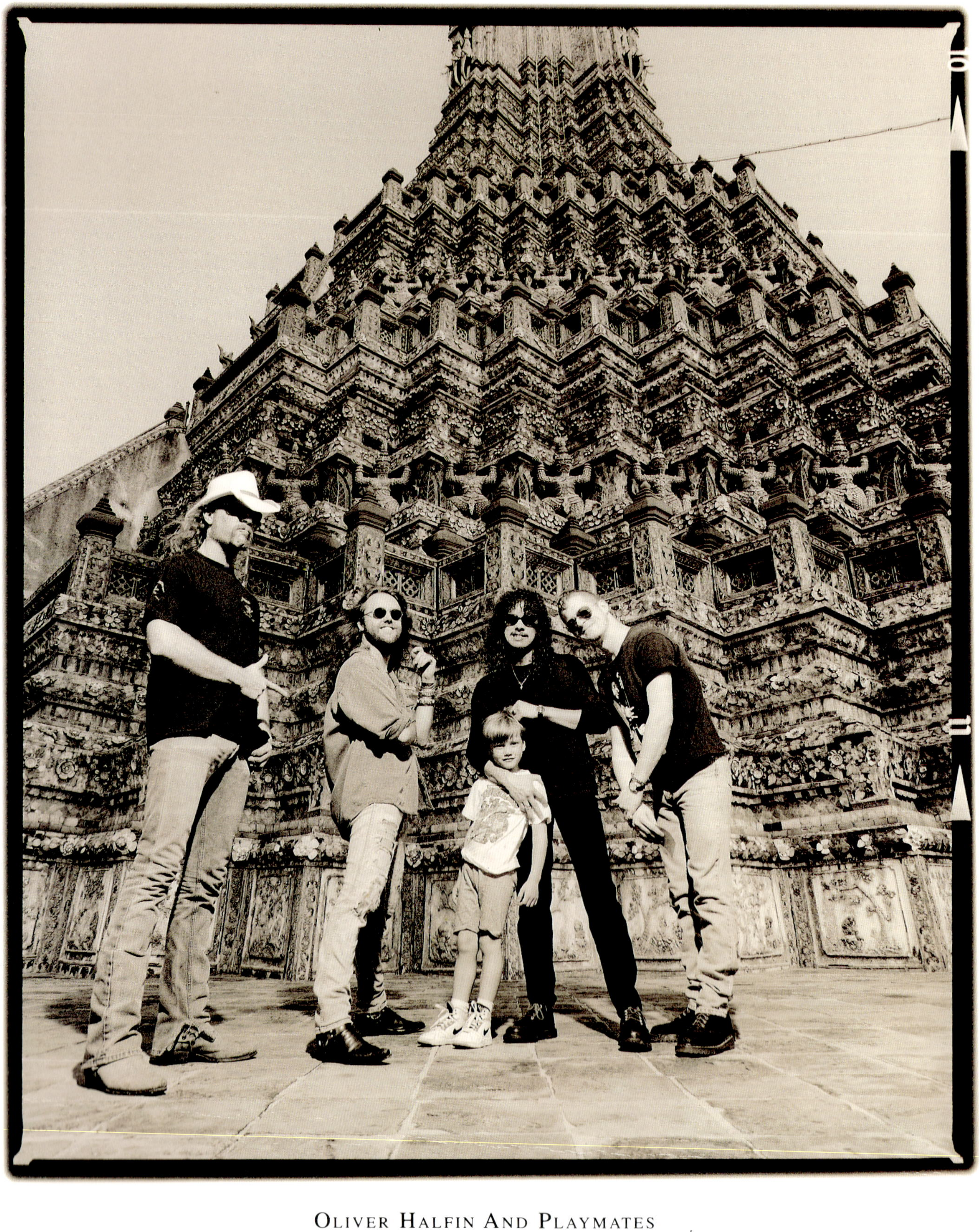

Oliver Halfin And Playmates
Wat Arun, Bangkok

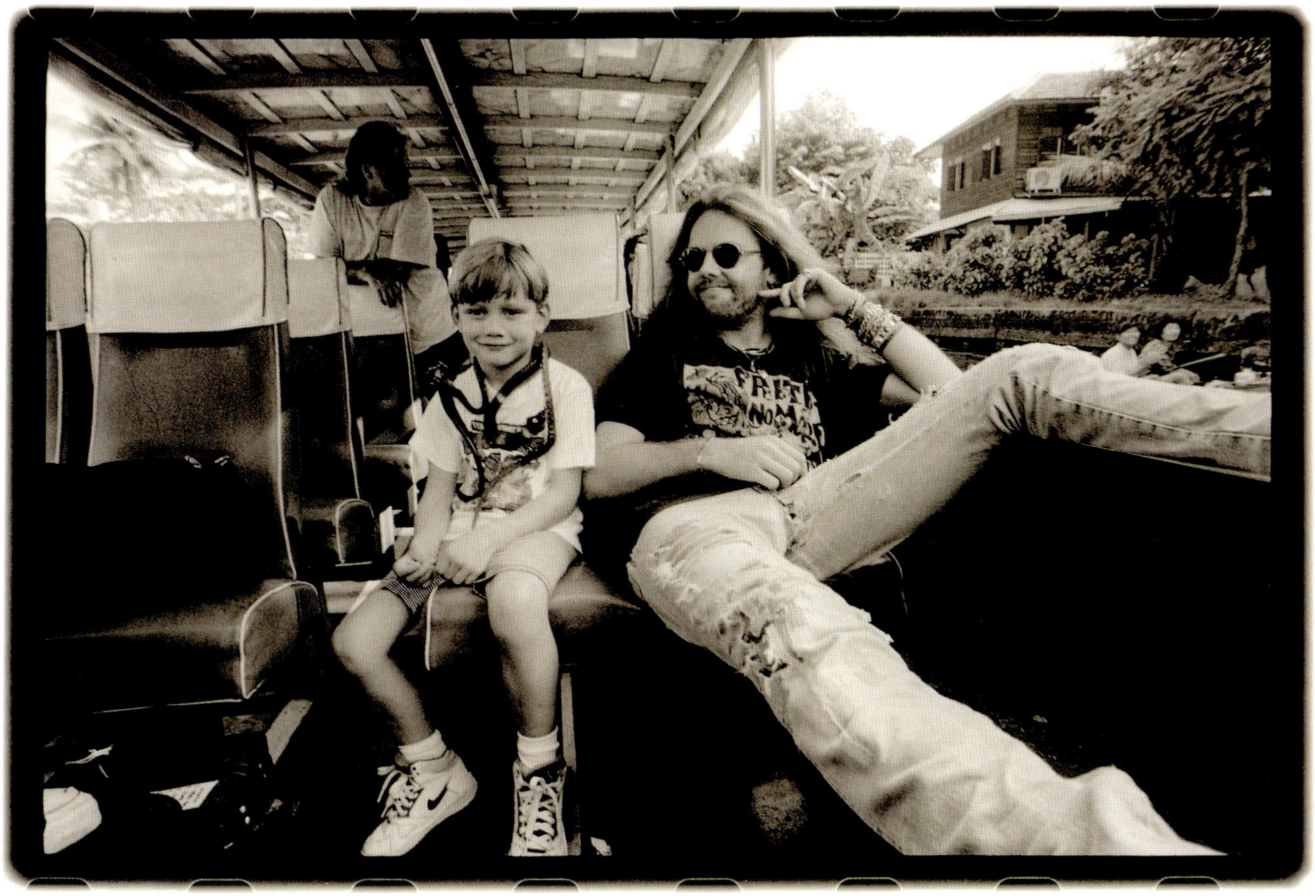

Oliver And Lars

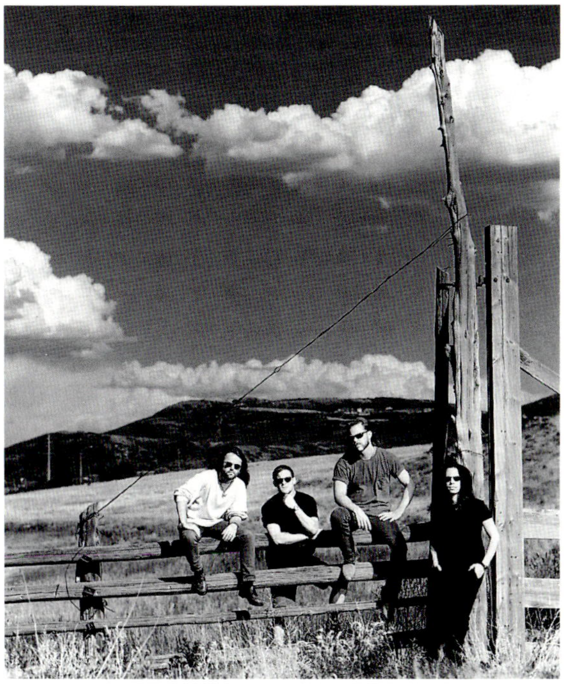

Metallica
Park City, Utah '94

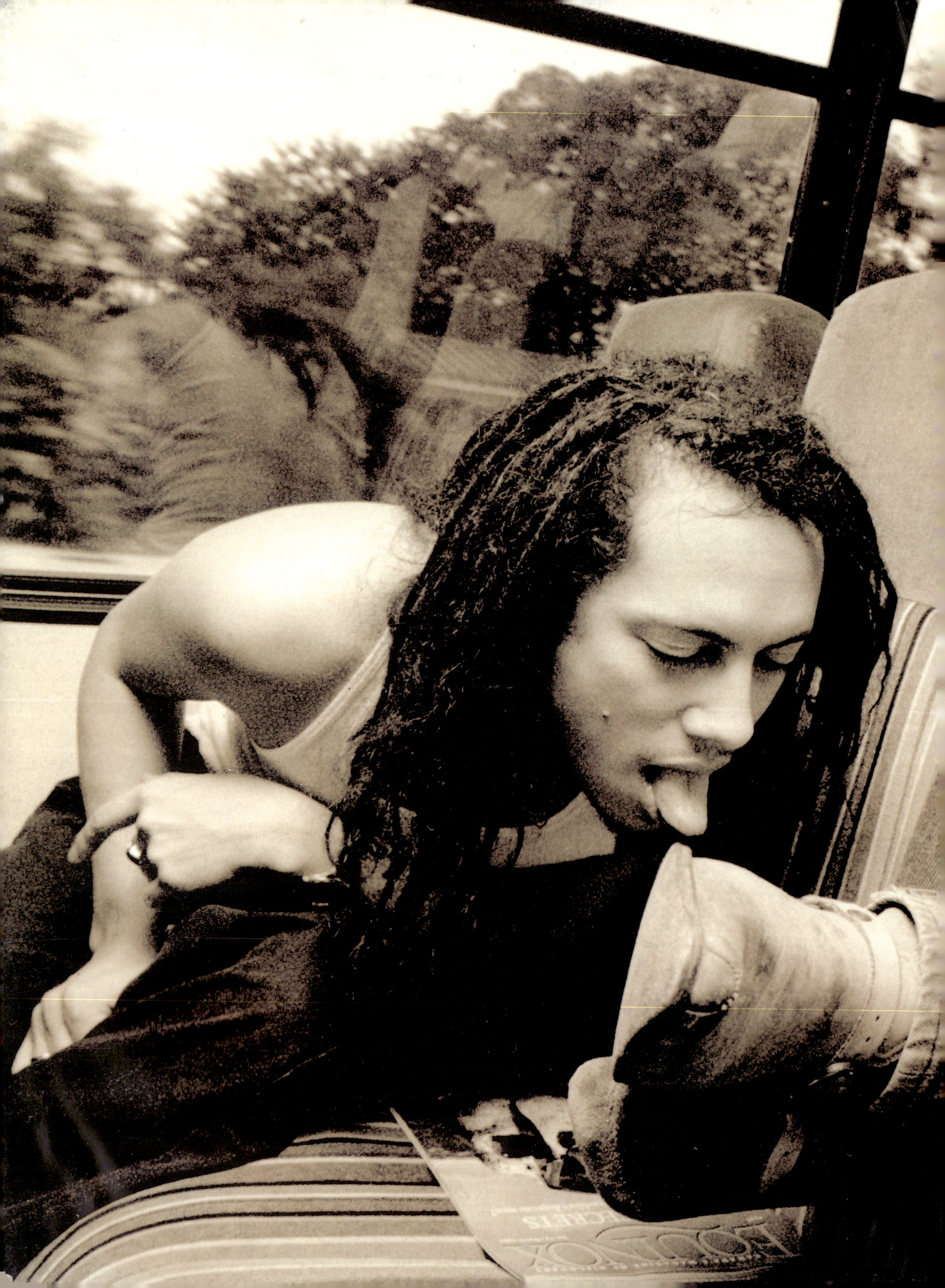

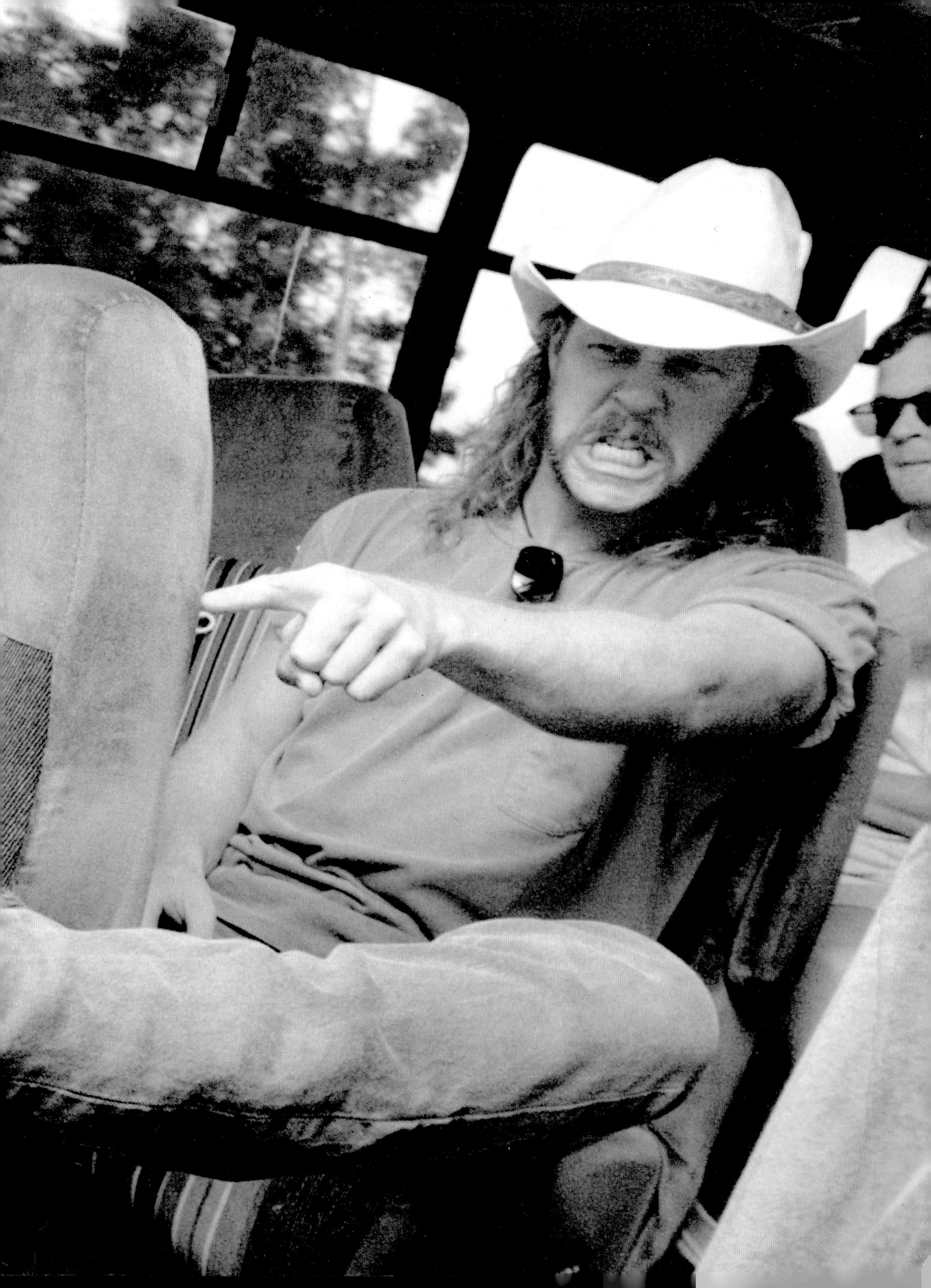

Lars and Kirk
Avenue of Death
Mexico City

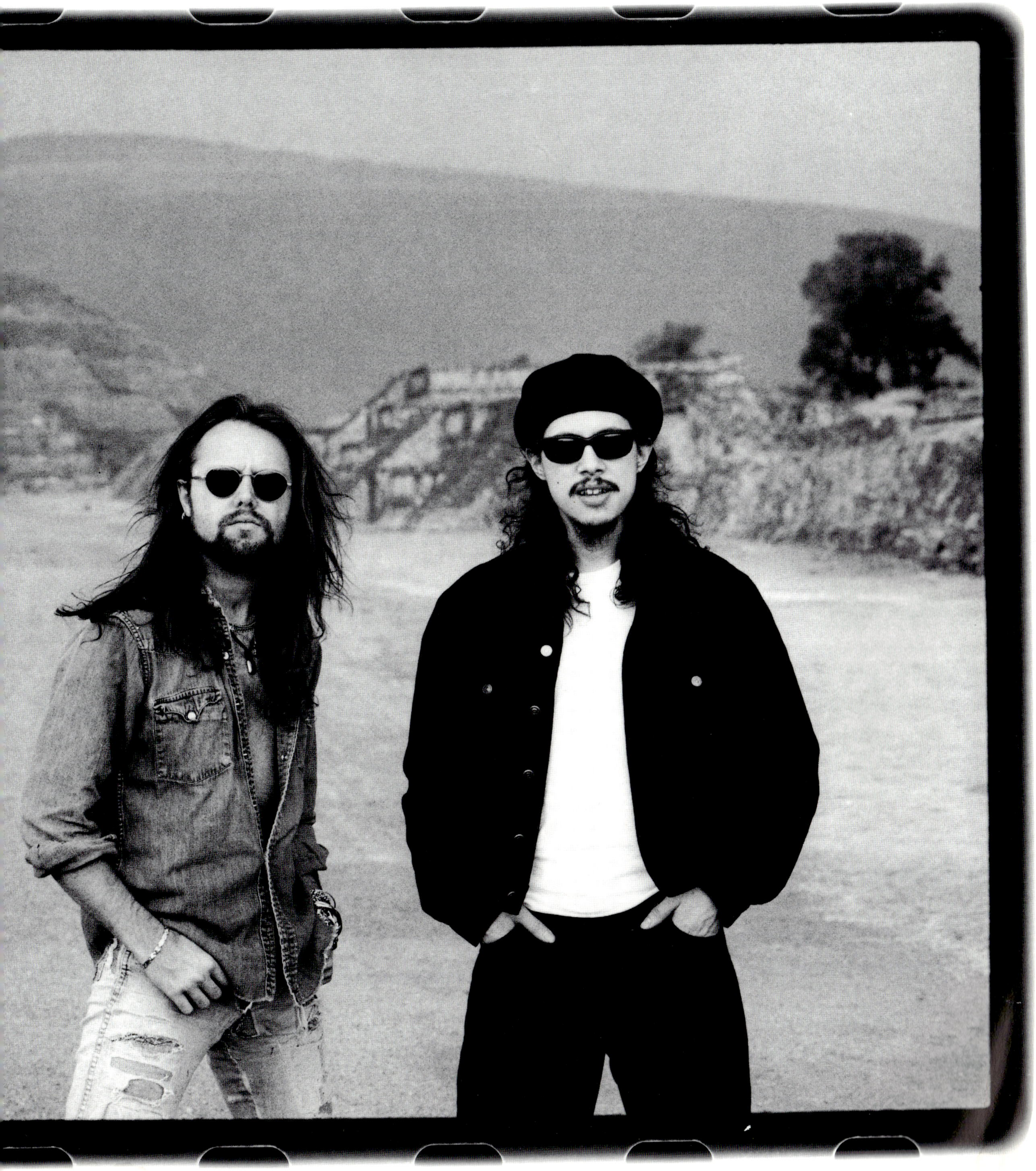

SOUNDGARDEN

SOUNDGARDEN
SYDNEY, '94

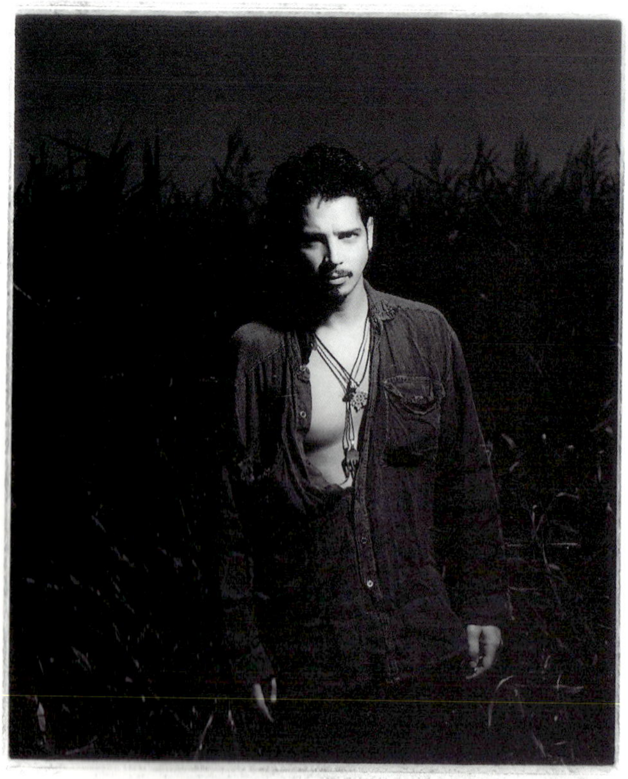

CHRIS CORNELL
MELBOURNE, '94

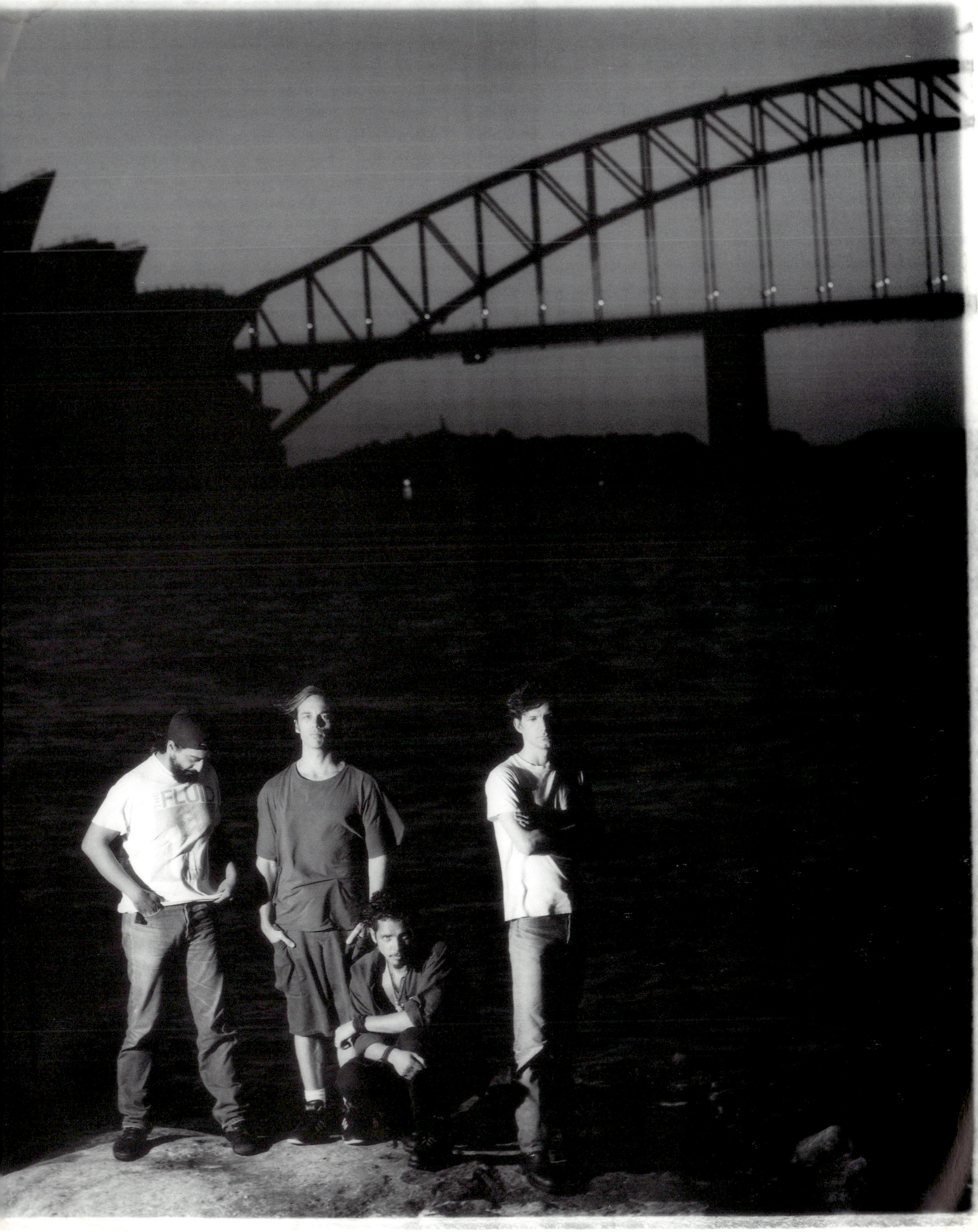

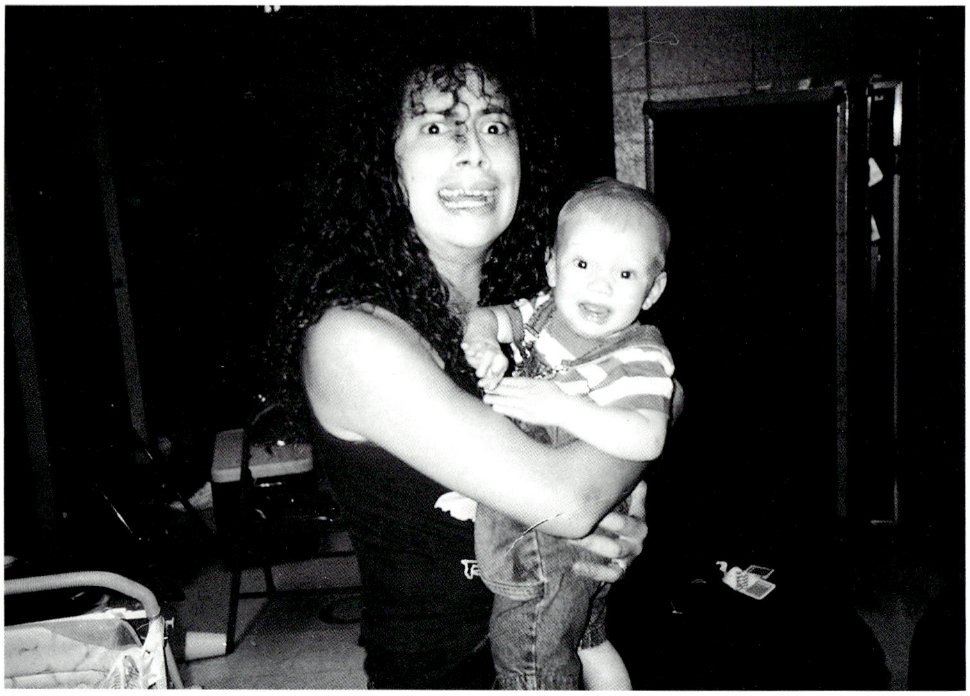

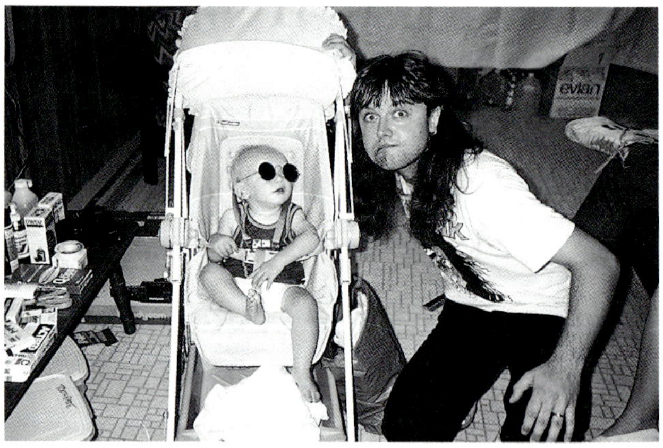

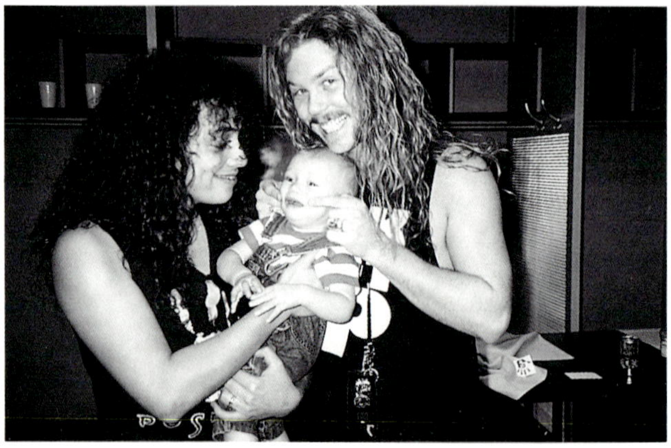

What About The Kids?

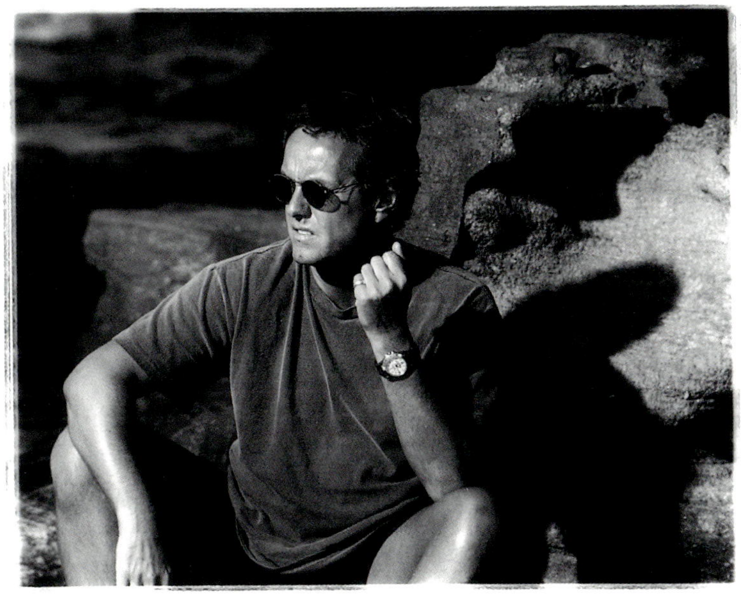

I wanted the book to be funny. It's meant to be more amusing than anything else. I want people to pick it up and be surprised. It's not some kind of high art trip. The pictures in this book weren't picked for their technical excellence or eye for detail. They are here because they tell stories. Some you might already know, others you almost certainly won't. All human life is here—from the sublime to the ridiculous. These are sideways glances that show a more human side to this business.

ROSS HALFIN

Hardcover ISBN 1-880985-21-7 Softcover ISBN 1-880985-22-5

First published 1996 by 2.13.61 Publications, Inc., Los Angeles.

Printed in Hong Kong.

2.13.61
P.O. BOX 1910 · LOS ANGELES · CALIFORNIA · 90078 · USA